THE IRISH HEALTH SYSTEM IN THE 21ST CENTURY

Edited by
Austin L. Leahy
Miriam M. Wiley

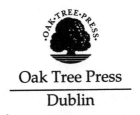

Oak Tree Press
Dublin

Oak Tree Press
Merrion Building
Lower Merrion Street
Dublin 2, Ireland
http://www.oaktreepress.com

A catalogue record of this book is
available from the British Library.

ISBN 1-86076-103-8

Printed in Britain by MPG Books, Bodmin, Cornwall

CONTENTS

PART FOUR: LEADERSHIP

LIST OF TABLES, FIGURES AND BOXES

ABOUT THE CONTRIBUTORS

Dr Ruth Barrington is Assistant Secretary of the Department of Health and Children. She is the author of *Health, Medicine and Politics in Ireland, 1900–1970* (IPA, 1987).

Dr Joseph Barry is Senior Lecturer in Public Health in the Department of Community Health and General Practice, Trinity College, Dublin, and a Specialist in Public Health Medicine for the Eastern Health Board.

Professor David Bouchier-Hayes MCh FRCS FRCSI is Chairman of the Department of Surgery at the Royal College of Surgeons in Ireland and Consultant Vascular Surgeon at Beaumont Hospital, Dublin.

Dr Denis Cusack FRCPI ACIArb is a Barrister-at-Law, Director and Senior Lecturer of the Division of Legal Medicine in University College Dublin, Director of the Medical Bureau of Road Safety, UCD, Kildare County Coroner and Founding Editor of the *Medico-Legal Journal of Ireland*.

Professor Ara Darzi FRCSI FRCS MD is Professor of Surgery in the Imperial College School of Medicine at St. Mary's Hospital, London.

Denis Doherty is Chief Executive Officer of the Midland Health Board and Director of the Office for Health Management.

Maeve Dwyer is Matron of the National Maternity Hospital, Holles Street, Dublin. She is a former President of the Irish Matrons Association and a Founder Fellow of the Faculty of Nursing (RCSI). She is a member of An Bord Altranais and the European Advisory Committee on the training of midwives.

Dr Tony Fahey is Senior Research Officer at The Economic and Social Research Institute.

Dr Yunnus Gul FRCSI is Senior Specialist Registrar of the Academic Surgical Unit at St. Mary's Hospital, London.

Professor Brian Lawlor is a Professor of Psychiatry for the Elderly at St. Patrick's and St. James's Hospitals and University of Dublin, Trinity College, Dublin.

Dr David McCutcheon is Chief Executive Officer of the recently merged Adelaide, Meath and National Children's Hospitals at the new hospital site in Tallaght. He is also a Lecturer in the Department of Community Health and General Practice at Trinity College Dublin.

Professor Andrew W. Murphy is Foundation Professor of General Practice at the National University of Ireland, Galway. He was previously the Senior Lecturer in the Department of General Practice at the Royal College of Surgeons in Ireland.

Professor Ciaran O'Boyle is a psychologist and pharmacologist and is currently Professor of Psychology and Chairman of the Department of Psychology in the Medical School of the Royal College of Surgeons in Ireland.

Jerry O'Dwyer is Secretary-General of the Department of Health and Children. A graduate of University College Dublin, he has worked in the Department since 1964.

Teresa O'Hara is Director of the Healthcare Management Centre at the Royal College of Surgeons in Ireland.

Donal O'Shea is Chairman of the Task Force on the Eastern Regional Health Authority and Chief Executive Officer of the North Eastern Health Board.

Dr Gregory Swanwick is a consultant psychiatrist with the Eastern Health Board and is President of the psychiatry section of the Royal Academy of Medicine in Ireland.

Peta Taaffe is Chief Nursing Officer in the Department of Health and Children. She is a Founder Fellow of the Faculty of Nursing, Royal College of Surgeons, a former President of the Irish Matrons Association and a member of the Commission on Nursing and An Bord Altranais.

FOREWORD

An Taoiseach, Mr Bertie Ahern TD

I am pleased to introduce this important book on the future direction of the Irish health services. It brings together many of the key contributors to health policy in recent years and offers valuable insights into the challenges facing us as the 21st century approaches.

In terms of quality and comprehensiveness, the Irish health and personal social services compare very favourably with services provided in other countries. Much of this is due to the quality of personnel and to the very high standards of care and service that they consistently provide. We owe a particular debt of gratitude to those who set about addressing the many challenges which they faced when developing the early health services. They did so generously, imaginatively and with innovation, at a time when resources were scarce and technologies were in their infancy.

Today, the service providers continue this work in what is now a very different and perhaps more challenging landscape. The Department of Health and Children celebrated its fiftieth anniversary last year. It has worked in partnership with service providers in an environment that is now substantially different to the one that existed in 1947. There are, of course, many challenges facing us in the health services today. These include:

- Responding in a timely way to the growing awareness among the public of health care issues, and their expectation and demand for high quality patient services;

- The rapidly growing complexity of the services to be provided, the range of educational skills required to deliver them, and the unique management challenges arising from those factors;

- The continuous development of medical technology, with corresponding increases in costs;

- The need to develop measures to evaluate and assess the overall effectiveness of emerging technology;

- The need to re-focus the services in light of the changing demographic profile of the population, particularly in light of an increasing number of people living longer;

- The continuing pressure to expand and develop worthwhile services in the area of personal social services and acute hospital care;

- The need to adopt an integrated approach across all sectors, to achieve health and social gain; and

- The continuing problem of distributing the finite resources for health services in an equitable, cost-effective and efficient manner.

As we prepare for the 21st century, I believe that we must preserve those features of our current system of which we are most proud, and that we should build upon them in order to promote the best possible health care system for 2000 and beyond. I believe that underlying all of our efforts should be the following principles:

- The patient must be placed at the centre of our system. We must never forget that the health services are there to serve and service the needs of patients and clients.

- We must continue to develop a quality culture in health care. This should be based on the principle of identifying optimum practices in treatment and care, and implementing them with the resources available.

- A strong sense of leadership will be needed in the health system to promote a clear direction for the century ahead. Both management and professionals must be encouraged to take a growing responsibility for the way in which health and personal social services are planned and delivered. Doctors, nurses and other health professionals have a vital role to play in this regard.

- Inevitably, the resources available for health care are finite. As pressure grows for more and more services, we must be prepared to evaluate the true outcome of treatments and to allocate money where it will achieve the greatest benefit. This is in keeping with the principles of health gain and social gain as identified in the Health Strategy, *Shaping a Healthier Future*.

- It is vital that we structure the Irish health system so that it can respond to the needs of the patients and clients. The restructuring that is currently in progress will be an essential element of our preparation for the health services of the 21st century.

The challenges which we face cannot be resolved by any one group in isolation. The partnership approach which is being pursued at national level through Partnership 2000 and, in the health sector, through the different working groups, committees and other forums, is the ideal way to reach consensus on the type and format of services we wish to see provided in the years ahead.

I welcome this book as a useful contribution to the debate about the future direction of our health services. It rightly deals with critical issues in the area of structures, management of quality, changing sectoral needs and the development of leadership by health professionals and managers.

Austin Leahy, Miriam Wiley and the distinguished contributors pose all the right questions and raise the right issues to stimulate an in-depth analysis of the way our health services should be, and the way our people want it to be in the 21st century. It will be highly relevant reading for everyone with an interest in health policy and health services.

Bertie Ahern TD
Taoiseach
September 1998

ACKNOWLEDGEMENTS

We would sincerely like to thank the authors who have given so generously of their time and expertise to make this publication possible. The contributors to this volume are all leaders in their respective fields and we are particularly appreciative of their support and commitment to standards of excellence when requested to honour very tight publication deadlines. The professionalism and expertise provided by Mr David Givens and Mr Brian Langan of Oak Tree Press has greatly facilitated the progression of this project from inception through to editing and publication, and their assistance is gratefully acknowledged.

INTRODUCTION

The new millennium approaches at a time of unprecedented economic prosperity. The success of Ireland's economic development can be attributed to many factors, not least of which is the emergence of a well-educated and healthy population. While the fate of current levels of prosperity may be difficult to predict, there is no disputing the importance of maintaining the highest achievable standards of health in order to safeguard the future wellbeing of Irish society.

This book provides guidance on how the Irish health system may be expected to develop in the coming decades. The new millennium will bring many challenges, some foreseen and others unexpected. What may be predicted with a reasonable degree of accuracy is that an expanding Irish population will bring ever-increasing expectations to bear on the level, range and scope of services required. If the Irish health system is to meet these challenges successfully, planning must be informed by past experience and based on modern developments in health care, both nationally and internationally.

With a view to assisting this process, the distinguished contributors to this volume were invited to explore the issues which would be expected to influence developments in the Irish health care system in the coming decades. As leaders in their respective fields, their views are based on a substantial body and range of experience. While it has been necessary to be selective regarding the issues given indepth consideration, this selectivity is in itself a positive feature, as it has ensured that the contributions are more concise and focused on the specific topic. By compiling these contributions in one volume, it is hoped to provide some indication of the pace and complexity of change that might be expected in the short to medium term. This should assist the anticipation of developments in the health system, particularly by those charged with the responsibility of ensuring that our health care system responds effectively to ever-expanding demands.

In this book, the discussion of the issues likely to influence the transition of the Irish health system into the 21st century centres around four main themes: the context of the health system; quality management; changing sectoral demands; and, finally, leadership.

In the first Part, the roots of the current structure of the Irish health system are clearly explored, together with an exposition of the many offshoots from this system since its inception. Chapter 1 outlines the current structure of the health system, and thereby provides a reference for all of the other chapters. The following two chapters discuss planned and potential changes in the organisation and structure of the Irish health system. The fact that a major review of the structure of this system is underway indicates that the importance of meeting future challenges has been recognised. These challenges may also be expected to apply substantial pressure on resources. The review of health system financing is therefore presented in Chapter 4 with a view to informing expectations regarding the level of support that might realistically be anticipated. There has been very substantial development in the political and legislative framework surrounding the health services in recent decades. The final chapter in Part One illustrates how the pace of development in this area may be expected to increase in complexity in the foreseeable future.

Pressure for future expansion in the range of available services will be accompanied by additional requirements for improvements in the quality of these services. In the second section, the demands of quality management are examined from a number of perspectives. In Chapter 6, the emergence of a quality culture within the health service is explored in some detail. This is followed, in Chapter 7, by a discussion of the requirements of risk management in pursuit of an operational strategy for quality. Quality of life assessment poses substantial challenges, both technically and methodologically. These techniques are discussed in Chapter 8 and their importance in estimating health gain is explained. The section on quality concludes with a discussion on how developments in medical technology may be assessed, using a number of emerging therapies as examples.

Part Three is concerned with an exploration of potential developments for specific areas and population groups. This section is introduced with a discussion of expected developments in the epidemiology of disease through to the next century. The demographic context in which these are likely to occur, particularly with regard to an ageing population, is outlined in some detail in Chapter 11. The elderly are the focus in the next chapter, which deals specifically with dementia. General practice and nursing are the subjects of the final two chapters of Part Three, which relate current and future challenges confronting professionals in both areas, and the likely effects these will have on the system in general.

The final Part concerns some important aspects of leadership in the Irish health services of the 21st century. The achievement of health and social gain is now considered an essential objective for this system and the first contribution in Part Four explores the associated requirements for the adaptation of health management structures. The discussion on this issue specifically addresses the importance of ensuring that structures adapt to needs and change accordingly. Chapter 16 concerns the integration and application of these skills in a multi-disciplinary and multi-sectoral context. There is a specific need for clinical staff to develop leadership skills and to participate in management at various levels. This is the focus of the final chapter, which specifically relates to management development for medical doctors.

The one point of certainty for any attempt at predicting the future is that there will be change. When the focus is health care, we can be assured that the pace of change will be rapid and far-reaching. The anticipation and management of change will be most productive when all parties to the process are well informed about the consequences of development. It is hoped that readers find this book interesting and relevant and that the contributions may be of assistance in informing the continued development of the Irish health system through to the next millennium.

PART ONE

The Context of the Irish Health System

1

CURRENT STRUCTURE OF THE IRISH HEALTH CARE SYSTEM — SETTING THE CONTEXT

Teresa O'Hara

INTRODUCTION

The health services in Ireland, like most other health care systems, face the challenge of providing accessible, high quality health care in an efficient and effective manner. This has to be achieved in the context of increased demands for service, increased use of high technology and expensive treatments, along with increases in the average length of life. How services are organised and delivered plays a key role in terms of their accessibility, quality and effectiveness. Often structural arrangements and the interfaces between organisations are the root causes of problems with service delivery, communication and access, with subsequent effects on the quality and outcomes of health care interventions. The solution to many service delivery problems often depends on first understanding the structural and organisational arrangements of the health system. The most quoted sentence from the comprehensive report of the Commission on Health Funding (Department of Health, 1989) highlights this issue by stating that

> the solution to the problem facing the Irish health services does not lie primarily in the system of funding but rather in the way that services are planned, organised and delivered.

This chapter provides an overview of the current organisation of services, concentrating on how the services are organised and managed at the central and local level and the core values that inform and guide policy development. It also highlights the recent policy reports and government statements that proposed changes, addressing the issues that cause fragmentation of service delivery and problems of service co-ordination. Subsequent chapters will look in more detail at the effects of implementing these proposals on the structure of the health system, the professionals delivering services and, most importantly, patients.

TYPE OF SYSTEM

The Irish health system is a mix of both public and private institutions and funders. Approximately 75 per cent is funded by the government, mainly through general taxation, and 25 per cent is funded mainly though voluntary health insurance premiums. Public health expenditure makes up approximately 20 per cent of government spending and in 1997 was 6.8 per cent of GNP. Private health expenditure accounts for nearly 25 per cent of health expenditure and approximately two per cent of GNP. Over 36 per cent of the population are eligible for all health services free of charge, based on means-testing of income. The rest of the population are entitled to public beds in public hospitals and if they wish they may avail of voluntary health insurance to cover private accommodation in public and private hospitals. Over 40 per cent of the population are enrolled in the two voluntary health insurance schemes.

CENTRAL ADMINISTRATION AND POLICY DEVELOPMENT

The organisation of public health and medical relief services in the nineteenth century provided the foundation on which the present health services developed (Department of Health, 1989). Since the end of the nineteenth century, the role of the state has also evolved from the provision of essential services funded locally to the poor, to playing a major role in the provision and funding of services, the regulation and setting of standards for inputs to the health system and, in recent times, an increasing emphasis on setting targets and objectives which will hopefully lead to the measurement of outcomes, along with outputs. In terms of making decisions on policy and service developments in the Irish context, "the power to decide what health services there will be and how they will be administered does not reside in any one person or institution" (Hensey, 1988). A combination of government, Department of Health and Children, advisory and executive agencies and voluntary organisations all play a role in service delivery and development, though their degree of power and influence varies. The rest of this chapter will look at the overall structure of the Irish health care system (Figure 1.1), the functions and roles of each of the parts and how they fit together in the context of the overall delivery of health care services.

Figure 1.1: Overall Structure of the Irish Health Care System

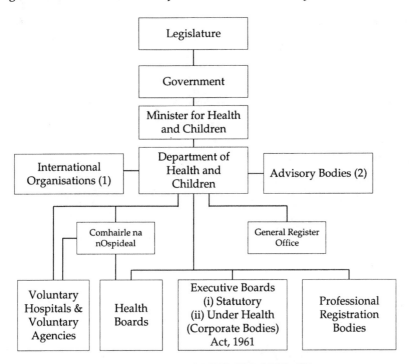

(1) WHO, UN, OECD, EU
(2) Food Safety Authority of Ireland
    National Ambulance Advisory Council
    Women's Health Council

Role of the Legislature and Government

The legal basis for the health services is contained in the acts passed by the Dáil and Seanad, and the actions of all organisations involved in administration must conform to these acts (Hensey, 1988). These acts are often preceded by a Green or White paper to stimulate debate and obtain the views of the public. As in the case of the other branches of the public services, decisions on the initiation of health legislation rests with the government (Hensey, 1988). The Minister for Health and Children first gets approval from cabinet colleagues, before placing a Bill before the Dáil. Amendments may be suggested by the Dáil or committees of the House, which may be incorporated into the Bill. After the Bill is passed by both Houses of the Oireachtas, and signed by the President, it then becomes an act. The acts governing the provision of the health services (e.g. the Health Acts of 1947, 1953 and 1970) do not lay down in detail how the services will operate but leave this to regulations made by the Minister, to guidelines and directives issued by the Department and to the decisions of the health boards and other executive agencies (Hensey, 1988).

Minister for Health and Children

The Minister for Health and Children is responsible for the strategic development and operation of the health services in accordance with legislation and government policy. The Minister initiates and formulates policies that may change the system and how it works for the benefit of the public (Hensey, 1988). The powers invested in the Minister include: the making of statutory regulations and orders; supervision of the activities of the health boards and other executive agencies; and control of the method of appointment, remuneration and the conditions of service of health personnel (Hensey, 1988). He or she does not have power to give directions on the eligibility of individuals for health services or how the services are to be made available to individuals. The recent policy documents from the Department suggest that the role of the Minister in terms of charting the strategic direction of the service will be promoted with much less involvement in the day-to-day running of the health services. It hopes to bring this about by reducing the number of agencies reporting directly to the Department, devolving executive work to other agencies and transferring the funding of voluntary agencies to health boards (Department of Health, 1997a, 1997b).

Secretary-General of the Department of Health and Children

The Secretary-General of the Department is the permanent head of the Department and is responsible for the overall administrative control of the Department, including staying within expenditure targets agreed by government, and seeing that the Minister's policies are implemented (Hensey, 1988). The Secretary-General is advised by a Management Advisory Committee in the formulation of policy proposals for the Minister. This consists of senior Department of Health officials, including the Chief Medical Officer, the Assistant Secretaries and the Division Directors.

Department of Health and Children

When the Ministers and Secretaries Act, 1924, set up the departments of the new state, it did not set up a separate Department of Health, but brought the health remit under the auspices of the Department of Local Government and Public Health (Barrington, 1987). Although the leader of the Labour Party at this time wanted to set up a separate Department of Health, this was rejected, and it wasn't until 1947 that a separate Department of Health was established under the Ministers and Secretaries (Amendment) Act, 1946 (Barrington, 1987). The Department has recently commemorated its fiftieth anniversary and in that time has seen major changes in the health status of the population as well as changes in the way services are organised and delivered (Robins, 1997). However, the Department also acknowledges that our life expectancy figures are still below those of most other countries in the EU and has made the reduction of cancer and cardiovascular disease, the two main causes of premature mortality in Ireland, a key objective of its strategy, *Shaping a Healthier Future* (Department of Health, 1994).

The titles of the Department and the Minister were changed in July 1997 to the Department of Health and Children and the Minister for Health and Children (Statutory Instrument No. 308 of 1997). This was a policy decision of the new Government that came into office in July 1997 and was done "to reflect the priority which the Government attaches to the improvement of services for children, particularly those considered to be at risk of abuse or neglect" as well as co-ordination of government policy in relation to children (Department of Health, 1998). There are also two Ministers of State under the Minister's remit. One has special responsibility for all services relating to children and the other has special responsibility for food safety and older people.

One of the key objectives of the Department of Health and Children is to support the Minister in the formulation, development and evaluation of health policy. It was the first department to be re-arranged according to the principles set out in the Report of the Public Services Organisation Review Group (1969). Each department was re-arranged with a separate policy-making "Aireacht" consisting of the Minister and top civil servants from executive offices and functions (Chubb, 1992). The executive functions were divided into staff and line units. The staff units consisted of planning, finance, organisation and personnel as well as, in the case of the Department of Health, the Chief Medical Officer and other professional staff. In recent years, the Department of Health and Children has been reorganised internally to strengthen its strategic role and to facilitate communications across functional and policy areas. The current Department of Health and Children comprises seven divisions, each representing a key area of its work. These are listed on the Department's organisation chart (Figure 1.2).

Objectives of the Department

The main objectives of the Department of Health and Children, as outlined in the 1997 Statement of Strategy are:

• To support the Minister in the formulation, development and evaluation of health policy and in the discharge of all other Ministerial functions;

Figure 1.2: Department of Health and Children: Organisation Chart (April 1998)

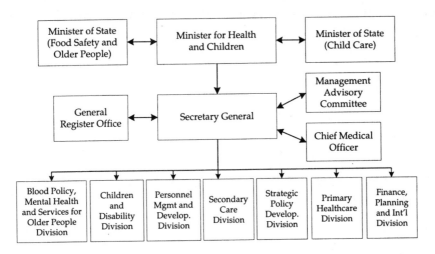

Source: Department of Health and Children

- To plan the strategic development of services, through partnership and consultation with health boards, the voluntary sector, other relevant government departments and other interests;

- To encourage the attainment of the highest standards of effectiveness, efficiency, equity, quality and value for money in the health delivery system;

- To strengthen accountability at all levels of the health services;

- To encourage the continuing development of a customer service ethos in the delivery of health services;

- To optimise staff performance, training and development;

- To represent the Irish interest in EU, WHO and international forums relating to health matters.

In order to achieve these objectives, the Department plans to "reposition" itself so that it will no longer be involved in the detailed management of services but play an increasing role in the strategic development of the services (Department of Health, 1997b). This fits in with the ethos of the Strategic Management Initiative in the civil service, focusing on a customer orientation and measurable results embedded in a strategic management process. It plans to do this by:

- Ending the direct funding by the Department of the voluntary hospitals and certain agencies and transferring funding of these agencies to the health boards;

- Devolving executive work to other agencies;

- Redefining its relationship with the agencies it funds by becoming less involved in operational matters and, through the mechanism of service planning, becoming more involved in measuring performance and evaluating services;

- Internally reorganising so that it will be able to take on this enhanced strategic role.

Executive Units within the Department

Within the Department there are three executive units:

1. *Office of the Registrar-General for Births, Deaths and Marriages*: This provides evidence of the occurrence and characteristics of vital events which feed into the compilation of vital statistics. These are necessary for the planning of both social and economic programmes.

2. *The Hospital Planning Office*: This unit co-operates with executive agencies in the design and building of hospitals and health facilities.

3. *Section for Superannuation Scheme for Voluntary Hospitals*: The most recent Statement of Strategy (Department of Health, 1997b) plans to transfer this responsibility to an appropriate agency. This is in line with the Department's philosophy of devolving executive functions to the appropriate agency and level.

Expert Groups and Working Parties

Practically all aspects of the health services have been covered by investigations by special working groups set up to investigate issues, advise on policy developments and make recommendations in key service areas. These expert groups make a significant contribution to the development of health policy and usually report on areas that have been identified as priorities by the Health Strategy or have come to the Department's attention as needing special attention or in-depth review. Below are listed some of the most recent working groups which reported in 1997 and 1998:

- Report of the National Task Force on Suicide (1998)

- Report of the Maternity and Infant Care Scheme Review (1997)

- Report of the Working Group on Bacterial Meningitis and Related Conditions (1997)

- Report of the Materials Management Advisory Group (1997)

- Enhancing the Partnership: Report of the Working Group on the Implementation of the Health Strategy in Relation to Persons with a Mental Handicap (1997).

Membership of these working parties usually consists of Department of Health officials and recognised experts in the service areas. Most of these groups also set up a process to obtain submissions for any groups, organisations or individuals who may have an input into the policy area before making final recommendations.

HEALTH SERVICE DELIVERY

The provision of health services in Ireland is the responsibility of five main types of bodies.

The Health Boards

Established under the Health Act, 1970 (discussed in next section).

The Voluntary Hospitals and other Voluntary Agencies

Voluntary agencies have played a key role in the provision of health and social services in Ireland. The Health Strategy recognises this role and states:

> The voluntary sector plays an integral role in the provision of health and personal social services in Ireland, which is perhaps unparalleled in any other country. Traditionally, voluntary organisations have been to the forefront in identifying needs in the community and developing responses to them. Their independence enables them to harness community support and to complement the statutory services in an innovative and flexible manner (Department of Health, 1994).

In the area of services to people with a mental handicap, they have been providing services since 1868 and are currently the major providers of services in this area. In the hospital sector, voluntary hospitals account for nearly 50 per cent of the hospital budget and are funded by the Department of Health and Children but run by both religious orders and lay boards of governors.

The proposed changes in recent policy reports will see the voluntary sector coming under the umbrella of the Health Board in terms of funding to facilitate regional service planning and funding. Up to now, most of these agencies have been directly funded from the Department of Health. The recent report, "Enhancing the Partnership", gives a detailed outline of how to facilitate "the smooth transfer of responsibility for funding of voluntary mental handicap agencies from the Department of Health to the health boards" (Department of Health, 1997c). Similar proposals will be necessary for the voluntary hospitals' integration into the new Eastern Regional Health Authority, which is one of the items on the agenda of the Task Force for the Eastern Region.

Specialist Bodies

These are established under specific acts, the most recent example being the Food Safety Authority of Ireland. Table 1.1 lists some of the main specialist bodies that perform a variety of advisory and service functions.

Table 1.1: Specialist Bodies

Irish Medicines Board Established in 1995 to take over the functions previously carried out by the National Drugs Advisory Board along with other functions.	*Main Functions:* • Responsible for the licensing of human and veterinary medicines, and the approval of clinical trials. • Acts as an advisory body to the Minister in relation to safety, control and regulation of medicines generally.
The Post Graduate Medical and Dental Board Established by the Medical Practitioners Act, 1978.	*Main Functions:* • To promote the development of postgraduate medical and dental education and training and co-ordinate such developments. • To advise the Minister for Health on all matters in relation to the development and co-ordination of this education and training. • To provide career guidance for registered medical practitioners and registered dentists.
Comhairle na nOspidéal Both an advisory and executive body set up under the Health Act, 1970.	*Main Functions:* • Statutory responsibility for the regulation of the number and type of appointments of consultant medical staff and senior registrars in hospitals and specifies qualifications for appointment of consultants. • Advises the Minister on matters relating to the organisation and operation of hospital services and publishes reports relating to such services. • 27 members appointed by the Minister for a five-year term of office. Over half of the members must be hospital consultants; the others officers of the Department of Health, voluntary hospitals and health board representatives.
Comhairle na Nimheanna Established by the Poisons Act, 1961.	Advises the Minister on the control of poisons.
Food Safety Authority of Ireland Established by the Food Safety Authority of Ireland (Establishment) Order, 1997.	Advises on issues relating to food safety, nutrition, food law and other matters related to the processing and sale of food.

National Council on Ageing and Older People Established by the National Council on Ageing and Older People (Establishment) Order, 1997.	Its main function is to advise the Minister on all aspects of the welfare of the elderly.
An Bord Uchtala (Adoption Board) Established by the Adoption Acts, 1952 to 1991.	This board decides on applications for adoption order and the registration of voluntary adoption societies.
Women's Health Council Established by the Women's Health Council (Establish-ment) Order, 1997.	To advise the Minister on all aspects of women's health.

Bodies Established under the Health (Corporate Bodies) Act, 1961

The Health (Corporate Bodies) Act, 1961, enables the Minister for Health to establish advisory and service agencies as bodies corporate, without the need for a separate Act of the Oireachtas each time. Many of these play a significant role in advising on health policy developments and the provision of those services which are more appropriately provided by a national organisation. Table 1.2 lists a number of these bodies and their functional remit.

Table 1.2: Bodies Established under the Health (Corporate Bodies) Act, 1961

Health Research Board Established in 1986, under the Health (Corporate Bodies) Act, 1961.	*Main functions*: • To promote, assist, commission or conduct medical, health and health services research and such epidemiological research as may appropriately or necessarily be carried out at national level. • To liase and co-operate with other research bodies in Ireland or elsewhere in promoting, commissioning or conducting relevant research. Its 1997 allocation from the Department of Health and Children was £3.8 million.

Blood Transfusion Service Board Established in 1965 under the Health (Corporate Bodies) Act, 1961, and replaced the National Blood Transfusion Association (set up in 1948).	*Main functions*: • To "organise and administer a blood transfusion service including the processing or supply of blood derivatives or other products and also including blood group and other tests in relation to specimens of blood received by the board" (1965, Order). • To make available blood and blood products. • To play a role in research, training and teaching in matters relating to blood transfusion and the preparation of blood products. It is headed jointly by a Chief Medical Consultant with clinical functions, and a Chief Executive Officer responsible for management issues. The Board consists of twelve members appointed by the Minister for Health who also nominates a Chairman from these members. The report on the Expert Group on the BTSB (Department of Health, 1995), set up to investigate the Hepatitis C incident, made a series of recommendations on how to improve the organisation and management of the service.
National Rehabilitation Board Established in 1967 under the NRB (Establishment) Order, Health (Corporate Bodies) Act, 1961.	*Main Functions*: • It provides occupational guidance, training and employment supports. • It provides a national hearing service for children and adults who qualify under the Health Act for the assessment of hearing loss • It also plays a role in improving public awareness of the needs and rights of people with disabilities and promotes a barrier-free environment for people with disabilities • It disseminates information on disability issues through its library, regional information centres and disability resource centres. The mission of the NRB is, on behalf of the state and in consultation with people with disabilities, to enable and empower them to live the life of their choice to their full potential.

Registration Bodies

The main professions — medicine, nursing, pharmacists, opticians and dentists — are each regulated under specific Acts by Bodies established under these Acts. These agencies uphold professional standards in order to protect the public from unqualified personnel or from negligence by qualified personnel. The relevant Acts, Bodies and functions of these bodies are outlined in Table 1.3.

Table 1.3: Registration Bodies

Medical Council	*Main Functions:*
Established under the Medical Practitioners Act, 1978.	• To prepare and establish a special register of medical practitioners. • To satisfy itself as to the suitability of medical education and training, including primary qualifications, clinical training and postgraduate education and training. • To inquire into the conduct of registered medical practitioners for alleged professional misconduct or fitness to engage in practice of medicine by reason of physical or mental disability. The Council consists of 25 members whose term of office is five years.
An Bord Altranais	*Main Functions:*
Established under the Nurses Act, 1950 and later reconstituted under the Nurse Act, 1985. It is the regulatory body of the nursing profession.	• To establish and maintain a register of nurses • To provide for the education and training of nurses and student nurses • To inquire into the conduct of alleged professional misconduct or alleged unfitness to engage in practice by reason of physical or mental disability. The board consists of 29 members whose term of office is five years — 17 are elected by nurses and 12 are appointed by the Minister.
Pharmaceutical Society of Ireland	*Main Functions:*
Established in 1875 by Act of Parliament to regulate the practice of pharmacy in Ireland.	• The education, examination and registration of pharmaceutical chemists, registered druggists and pharmaceutical assistants. • The enforcement of regulations relating to the sale and distribution of poisons and controlled preparations. • The administration of the Pharmacy Acts, 1875–1977.

Dental Council	*Main Functions:*
Established under the provisions of the Dentists Act, 1985.	• To promote high standards of professional education and conduct among dentists. • To establish and maintain a register of dentist and dental specialists. • To satisfy itself at to the adequacy, suitability and standards of dental education provided by training institutions in the state. • To inquire into the fitness of a registered dentist to practise on the grounds of alleged professional misconduct or alleged unfitness to practise by reason of physical or mental disability. • To establish schemes with the consent of the Minister for different categories of auxiliary dental worker. In 1995, there were 1,609 dentists and 113 dental hygienists registered with the council.

HEALTH BOARDS

The health boards have a statutory responsibility for administering the services provided for in health legislation and by ministerial initiative. The establishment of the health boards in 1971 brought about one of the biggest changes in the way that services are organised: "the change from a locally controlled and locally financed system to an increasingly centralised and centrally financed health system" (Barrington, 1987). When the Department of Health was established, the administrative structures of local government, consisting of county councils and county boroughs, were thought to be the most effective mechanisms for the administration of public-health-related functions (Department of Health, 1997). By the 1960s, it became clear that the county as a unit was too small, especially for the planning and delivery of acute services. The 1966 White Paper outlined the reasons for the necessity for regionalisation of health services, which led to the passing of the Health Act, 1970. On 1 April 1971, the administration of the health services became the responsibility of eight health boards, each covering a number of counties (Section 4 (1) of the Health Act 1970). In setting up the health boards, consideration was given to the size of the area, the population of the area, and local government planning and development (Curry, 1993). The eventual size of the eight health boards was the result of a compromise based on common sense rather than on science (Hensey, 1988). The population of each health board currently ranges from just over 200,000 in the Midland Health Board to nearly 1.3 million or 36 per cent of the total population who reside in the Eastern Health Board region. Table 1.4 gives details of the population served by each board and the changes over the last 25 years. The largest increase in numbers has taken place in the Eastern Health Board, which has implications for the capacity of current services, as well as taking into account the many tertiary services located in this health board area. The density of the population in each health board ranges from 257 per sq. km in the Eastern Health Board to 25–36 per sq. km in the Western Health Board. Access to services and the appropriate level of service to provide in rural and less densely populated areas are factors which impinge on service organisation and delivery.

Health Board Governance

Section 4 (2) of the Health Act, 1970, specifies in broad terms the constitution of each health board and how the boards are to be managed. Health board meetings are usually held on a monthly basis and are open to the press. The membership of health boards is a combination of three main interest groups:

- **Elected representatives from county councils and borough councils.** These representatives account for more than half the members. Making this group the largest representative group on the boards was envisaged as one way of keeping the boards responsive to local interests (Dooney and O'Toole, 1992). The same philosophy is guiding current proposals on membership of the proposed Area Councils in the new Eastern Regional Health Authority, which will replace the Eastern Health Board (Department of Health, 1997a).

Table 1.4: Population and Percentage Distribution for each Health Board Area, 1971–96

	1971		1986		1991		1996	
Eastern	990,491	33.3%	1,232,238	34.8%	1,245,225	35.3%	1,295,939	35.7%
Midland	178,098	6.0%	207,944	5.9%	202,984	5.8%	205,542	5.7%
Mid-Western	269,804	9.1%	315,435	8.9%	310,728	8.8%	317,069	8.7%
North-Eastern	245,540	8.2%	302,035	8.5%	300,183	8.5%	306,155	8.4%
North-Western	186,979	6.3%	212,745	6.0%	208,174	5.9%	210,872	5.8%
South-Eastern	328,604	11.0%	384,974	10.9%	383,188	10.9%	391,517	10.8%
Southern	465,665	15.6%	536,894	15.2%	532,263	15.1%	546,640	15.1%
Western	312,267	10.5%	348,328	9.8%	342,974	9.7%	352,353	9.7%
	2,978,258	100.0%	3,540,643	100.0%	3,525,719	100.0%	3,626,087	100.0%

Source: Department of Health Statistics, 1997.

- **Professional Representatives.** These are mainly officers of the health board and include doctors, nurses, dentists and pharmacists, elected by their peers.

- **Nominees of the Minister for Health (three on each board).** Initially these nominees represented excluded professional groups, but increasingly they tend to represent the consumers of health services (Dooney and O'Toole, 1992).

The Eastern Health Board, the largest health board, has 38 members. These include: 13 professionals (nine medical practitioners, one dentist, one nurse, one psychiatric nurse and one pharmacist); three ministerial appointees; and 22 public representatives.

The 1994 Health Strategy identified several weaknesses in the structure of the Health Boards. These included:

- A lack of clarity with regard to the respective roles and responsibilities of health boards and their chief executive officers;

- Inadequate accountability within the structures;

- Over-involvement by the Department of Health in the detailed management of the services.

The Health (Amendment) Act, 1996, has as its primary purpose to tackle these weaknesses by strengthening the financial accountability of the boards and clarifying the respective roles of the members of the health boards and their chief executive officers.

Section 2 of the Act specifies very clearly the manner in which health boards are to carry out their functions. These include:

- **Resource allocation**: securing the most beneficial, effective and efficient use of whatever resources are available to the board;

- **Inter-organisational co-operation**: co-operating with voluntary bodies providing services to people in the health board area;

- **Multi-sectoral co-operation**: co-operating with and co-ordinating its activities with those of other health boards, local authorities and public authorities who perform functions related to the health of the population of the health board;

- **Implementing government policy**: giving due consideration to the policies and objectives of the Government or any Minister of the Government in so far as they may affect or relate to functions of the health board.

These new accountability measures go into effect in 1998 and will be monitored closely by the Department of Health, especially through evaluation of the Health Board's Service Plans.

Service Planning

Section 6 of the Health (Amendment) Act, 1996, specifies that each board must submit a service plan to the Minister on an annual basis. Service planning is part of the strategic planning ethos emphasised in the government's Strategic Management Initiative and the Health Strategy of 1994. Section 6.2 of the Health (Amendment) Act, 1996, states that these plans should "include a statement of the services to be provided by the health board and estimates of the income and expenditure of the board for the period to which the plan relates", as well as taking account of the financial limits determined by the Minister for Health and Children. It is hoped that service plans will also identify priority areas — both unmet needs and changing patterns of needs — and eventually incorporate performance measures of health outcomes.

The Task Force Report on the Eastern Region envisages that service planning will play a pivotal role in enhancing the funding and partnership arrangements in the regions. It recommends that the major acute hospitals and the proposed Area Health Councils should negotiate service agreements with the Authority for a period of three to five years. It proposes that these plans should include certain common elements such as: the quantum of service to be provided; effectiveness; efficiency; quality; equity; access; appropriateness of care and responsiveness to the public (Department of Health, 1997a). It is hoped that the use of service planning will provide transparency, equity and fairness to the funding of both statutory and voluntary services in the new Eastern Authority.

The Department of Health and the CEOs of the Health Boards have both set up working groups to devise a framework for formulating service plans. They hope to come up with a joint agreement on what should be the general format and content of service plans and to provide a set of guidelines to all those involved in service planning.

Management of the Health Boards

The McKinsey Report (1970) recommended a management structure for the health boards, which was subsequently adopted. This was based on the concept of a management team directed by the Chief Executive Officer and supported by the functional officers and the programme managers (Figure 1.3). This team now includes the new Directors of Public Health, who, it is hoped, will make a major contribution to the service planning activities of the health board, in terms of measuring health needs and evaluating outcomes, as well as giving advice on the public health dimensions of service delivery. The Chief Executive Officer of the board is responsible for the day-to-day administration of the services including personnel matters, as well as advising the health board. The Chief Executive Officer has a limited range of decision-making power in deciding on eligibility of individuals for services.

For administration purposes, most of the health boards are divided into divisions or programme areas. These are:

- Community Care Services

- General Hospital Services

- Special Hospital Services.

While some of the smaller boards amalgamate the two hospital programmes, the Eastern Health Board has expanded and refined the number of programme areas, each with a separate programme manager. The Eastern Health Board now has five programme managers in the following areas:

Figure 1.3: Health Board Management

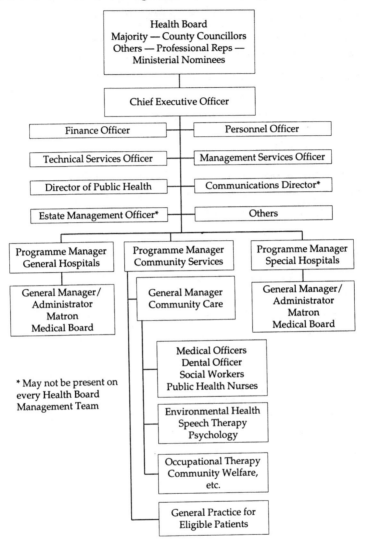

- Community Services Programme
- Acute Hospital Services and the Elderly
- Health Promotion, Mental Health, Addiction and Social Development
- Services for Persons with Disabilities
- Children and Families Programme.

It is not yet clear how these programme areas will be integrated into the new organisational arrangements for the Eastern Regional Health Authority. The responsibilities of the programme managers include service planning, taking into account service needs and resource requirements as well as setting targets for service development. Table 1.5 gives a broad overview of the type of services which are provided under the three main programme areas in all health boards.

Table 1.5: Health Board Programme

Programme Area	Type of Service
Community Care	General Practitioner Services
	Child Care and Family Support Services
	Dental, Ophthalmic, Aural Services
	Maternity and Infant Care Scheme
	Supplementary Welfare Services
	Services for the Elderly
	Public Health Nursing Services: Family Planning/Pregnancy Counselling/ Women's Health Services/Hepatitis C
	Environmental Health Services
	Care of Deprived Children
	Services for Travellers
	Services for People with Physical/ Sensory Disabilities
	Community Drugs Schemes
Special Hospital	Adult Psychiatric Services
	Old Age Psychiatry Services
	Mentally Handicapped Services
	Alcoholism Services
	Addiction Centres
General Hospitals	Medical, Surgical Hospitals
	Maternity Hospitals
	Out-patient Clinics
	Ambulance and Transport Services
	Pharmacy Services

Development of the General Medical Services Scheme

The general practitioner services in Ireland have their roots in the Poor Relief (Ireland) Act, 1851, which placed a duty on the Irish Poor Law Commissioners to provide dispensaries and appoint medical officers. Although it facilitated the development of medical care in rural Ireland and made up for the deficiencies of the infirmaries of the time, the quality of the care, as well as the conditions that the doctors worked in, were not always good (Hensey, 1988). Although there were some minor changes in service delivery over the years in terms of eligibility and selection of doctors to work in the system, it wasn't until the 1966 White Paper that there were proposals to change the service radically (Hensey, 1988). One of the main criticisms of the service that the White Paper tried to address was that it led to the development of a two-tier system with patients using the dispensary service having no choice of doctor as well as being separated from private medical patients. This eventually led to the introduction of the General Medical Services Scheme in 1972, established jointly by the eight health boards, which provided for a choice of doctor and pharmacist for those eligible for the services based on means-testing of income. A further review of the service in 1984 eventually led to the introduction in 1989 of a system of capitation payments and superannuation (Department of Health, 1984). In recent years, other planning developments have included the setting up of a General Practice Development Fund which has supported the development of General Practice Units in the Health Boards and support of continuing education, information technology, premises development and services provision.

Hospital Services

Hospital services account for 50 per cent of health expenditure. Public acute hospitals are classified into two types:

Health Board Hospitals

These are financed by state funds and administered by the health boards under their general hospital care programme.

Public Voluntary Hospitals

These hospitals originated in the early years of the eighteenth century, established by lay people and in later years by religious orders. Their development was almost entirely confined to city areas such as Dublin and Cork, as they depended on funding from commercial and professional classes who were mainly found in urban areas (Department of Health, 1968). Today, they are now owned and operated by both religious orders and lay boards of governors. They are also largely financed by state funds, having a direct funding relationship with the Department of Health. Three of these hospitals in the Dublin area have recently amalgamated and moved to a new site in Tallaght in June 1998. This is part of a rationalisation programme for the acute hospital sector which was first proposed in 1968 as part of a national plan for the development of hospital services in Ireland (Department of Health, 1968). The proposed changes in the Eastern region plans to transfer the funding of these hospitals from the Department of Health to the new Eastern Regional Health Authority. Table 1.6 gives an overview of the numbers of public voluntary and health board hospitals in each of the health board regions and the average length of stay and number of beds. The number of inpatient beds in 1996 was 11,937, compared to the 1985 figure of 14,868. Reductions in length of stay and the increased use of day-care have contributed to the decrease in beds, as have hospital closures in the late 1980s.

Table 1.6: Publicly Funded Acute Hospitals, 1996

	Number of Hospitals	Average No. of Inpatient Beds Available	Average Length of Stay (Days)	Number of Day Cases
Eastern	25	4,970	7.5	127,469
Midland	3	468	5.4	6,726
Mid-Western	6	783	6.2	14,826
North-Eastern	5	911	6.0	10,061
North-Western	3	668	5.4	16,308
South-Eastern	6	1,109	5.3	13,352
Southern	9	1,795	6.1	31,508
Western	5	1,233	6.4	13,658
Total	62	11,397	6.5	233,098

PRIVATE HEALTH SERVICES

The private sector accounts for approximately two per cent of the GNP or 25 per cent of total expenditure on the health services. The private hospital sector receives no direct government funding and is run on a non-profit basis. There are 20 private hospitals, most of whom are members of the Independent Hospital Association (IHA). This organisation was originally formed in 1992 to lobby for the interests of private hospitals with the main health insurer at the time, the Voluntary Health Insurance (VHI). In recent times they are also looking at costing and accreditation systems suitable for this sector.

Until 1996, the VHI was the principal private health insurer, giving it considerable power when negotiating contract agreements with service providers. The Health Insurance Act of 1994 opened up the market for health insurance, bringing BUPA into the market in 1996. The 1994 Act retained certain features of the system such as community rating, open access and lifetime cover. Insurers are also required to provide a minimum level of benefits, and a risk equalisation scheme is part of the regulations. However, the VHI are still the major health insurer with nearly 1.4 million subscribers, with only 60,000 subscribers signing up with BUPA. The lack of competition in the Irish market has been attributed to the state ownership of VHI, giving it a dominant position, and the current lack of an independent regulator, other than the government of the insurance market.

REAPPRAISAL OF THE DIRECTION AND ORGANISATION OF THE HEALTH SERVICES, 1986–94

Since the late 1980s, there has been a distinct emphasis in many of the working groups and policy reports on obtaining an understanding of how the organisation of the system hinders or facilitates service delivery. Table 1.7 highlights the significant working groups, reports and statements that contributed to the reappraisal of the organisation and strategic outlook of the service over this time period. This section looks at the strategic and structural initiatives proposed by these working groups and reports and more importantly what problems or issues they hoped to address in terms of optimum service delivery.

Table 1.7: Major Milestones in Strategic Direction and Re-organisation of the Irish Health Services, 1986–97 — Reports and Ministerial Statements

1986	Health: the Wider Dimensions
1989	Commission on Health Funding
1990	Dublin Hospital Initiative Group (Kennedy Reports)
1991	Minister's Statement on the Restructuring of the Eastern Region
1994	Shaping a Healthier Future
1996	Minister's Statement on the Restructuring of the Eastern Region
1997	Statement of Strategy: Department of Health & Children
1997	Interim Report of the Task Force on the Eastern Regional Health Authority
1997	Enhancing the Partnership: Report of the Working Group on the Implementation of the Health Strategy in Relation to Persons with a Mental Handicap
1998	Strategy Statement 1998–2001: Working for Health and Well-Being

1986 — Health: the Wider Dimensions

In 1986, the Department of Health published a consultative statement on its policy direction, "Health: the Wider Dimensions", which marked the beginning of a reappraisal of the direction and orientation of the health services. Its main purpose was to ascertain the Irish position with regard to implementing the WHO objectives in its initiative, "Health for All by the Year 2000". It was the first attempt at setting a direction for the health services and placing the services in relation to meeting health-related targets. Its broad view of health policy meant that a "considerable reorientation" in the traditional perception of health and health services was needed, with an emphasis on multi-sectoral planning and health promotion.

1989 — Report of the Commission on Health Funding

The Commission on Health Funding was set up in 1987:

> to examine the financing of the health services and to make recommendation on the extent and source of the future funding required to provide an equitable, comprehensive and cost-

effective public health service and on any changes in administration which seem desirable for that purpose.

Its terms of reference emphasised the funding of the service, but the Report of the Commission on Health Funding is most remembered for its analysis of the key faults in the organisation of health services which led to the fragmentation of service delivery. These included:

- Confusion of the political process which should decide the type, quality and funding of the service and the executive function which should be responsible for the day-to-day management of the services;

- Imbalance between national decision-making, which should be concerned with broad planning, and local decision-making, which should be concerned with the details;

- No evaluation of the effectiveness, efficiency or quality of the service;

- Inadequate accountability;

- Insufficient integration of related services;

- Inadequate representation of service users.

The subsequent policy reports and structural changes had these six deficiencies in mind when they set about making changes in service delivery and organisation.

1990 — Dublin Hospital Initiative Group: "Kennedy Reports"

This review group, chaired by Professor David Kennedy, was set up in 1990 to improve the co-ordination of hospital services and the integration of hospital and other services in the Dublin area. It made a number of recommendations in relation to management of hospital workload, but one of its key recommendations was in relation to restructuring the Eastern Health Board with the creation of a single new authority to replace the Eastern Health Board, with five area units reporting to it. In order to plan for service delivery and development, it recommended that the Department of Health should be less involved in the direct management of services and take a greater role in policy and strategic issues. It also advocated the development of service contracts with voluntary agencies to be administered by the area units to facilitate co-ordination of services.

1991 — Minister's Statement on the Restructuring of the Eastern Region

The importance of this statement was that it signalled the adoption by the government of the recommendations contained in the Kennedy reports with regard to the establishment of a new authority to replace the Eastern Health Board. The principles on which this re-organisation was based were: devolution of responsibility to the lowest level; improvement of co-ordination between hospital and community-based services; clearer definition of roles; and a constant search for greater efficiency. The Minister also acknowledged the key role played by voluntary organisations and the need for the new authority to enter into funding agreements with the voluntary agencies. It was also important in terms of signalling the commitment of successive governments to the restructuring of the service and avoiding politicisation of the issue.

1994 — Health Strategy: *Shaping a Healthier Future*

In April 1994, one of the most significant health policy and planning documents, *Shaping a Healthier Future*, was launched. Its main focus was the re-orientation and reshaping of the health services so that improving people's health and quality of life became the primary and unifying focus of the health services. It put forward three principles which should underpin all future service developments:

- **Quality**: both technical quality and the consumer's perception of quality;

- **Equity**: access according to need rather than ability to pay or geographic location, as well as addressing the variations in health status of different groups in society;

- **Accountability**: legal and financial responsibility needs to be taken; those providing the service should take responsibility for the achievement of the agreed objectives.

It outlined three dimensions to this re-orientation:

- **The Service Dimension**: increased emphasis on health promotion and disease prevention, appropriate provision of treatment and continuity of care, backed up by information and evaluation and linkages between services;

- **The Framework**: the need to get the organisational and management structure of the system right to ensure that it supports the delivery of the services;

- **The Participants**: while it recognised that one of the strengths of the Irish system was the well-qualified, committed and caring staff, the document also recognised that the patient's or client's perspective was integral to service delivery, as was having staff with the proper training and education.

Since the Strategy was launched, there have been further policy documents produced which tie in with the implementation of programmes to meet the targets and objectives of *Shaping a Healthier Future*. These include:

- 1995 — Health Promotion Strategy

- 1996 — National Policy on Alcohol

- 1996 — Management Development Strategy for the Health and Personal Social Services

- 1996 — Cancer Strategy and a Cancer Action Plan

- 1996 — Minister's statement on the Restructuring of the Eastern Region

- 1997 — Plan for Women's Health.

Although there were many changes in government at this time, the consistent approach in health policy initiatives highlighted a political

consensus on the strategic development of the health services. Another underlying trend in many of these reports is a changing role for
the Department of Health: more involvement in policy development
and strategic planning and less involvement in the detailed management of the services, with devolvement of decision-making to the
most appropriate level.

1996 — Minister's Statement on the Restructuring of the Eastern Region

The purpose of this Ministerial Statement was to announce government approval for the proposal to establish an Eastern Regional
Health Authority. It again reiterated the political consensus in terms
of the restructuring, as well as adding some key dimensions on representation and management of the authority. It stated that:

- Public representatives will hold the majority on the new Authority;

- The Authority will also include persons drawn from the voluntary hospitals, mental handicap agencies and other voluntary
bodies;

- The Authority will be managed through three Area Health
Councils, with Area Managers.

A Task Force was also established to work out the detailed organisational and administrative arrangements required for the transition to
the new structures.

1997 — Interim Report of The Task Force of the Eastern Regional Health Authority

This was the first report from the group set up by the Minster in November 1996 to oversee and manage the implementation of the proposed restructuring. The key strategic and structural initiatives
proposed by this group included:

- The Eastern Health Authority would have no management role
in the direct delivery of services. Its role would consist of the
identification of the health and social needs of the population;

planning the services for the region; allocation of funding; and commissioning for service provision with service providers based on service agreements.

- The Area Health Councils would perform the following role: identify health needs and priorities in its area; ensure that services agreements with the Centre are adhered to; co-operate with voluntary providers; monitor the overall provision of health and social services in the area.

1997 — Statement of Strategy: Department of Health and Children

This was the Department of Health and Children's response to the Strategic Management Initiative in the civil service, in terms of outlining its own mission statement, objectives and "new" role for the Department. The mechanisms it put forward to enable it to carry out its new role included the devolvement of executive work, the redefinition of relationships with funded agencies, with a focus on performance measurement, services evaluation and internal reorganisation, as depicted in Figure 1.2.

1998 — Working for Health and Well-Being: Strategy Statement 1998–2001

The latest Department of Health and Children Strategy Statement builds upon the Strategy Statement of 1997 and the strategic direction mapped out for the health services in *Shaping a Healthier Future* in 1994. It highlights the importance of the repositioning of the Department in terms of meeting its objectives and the challenges that recent initiatives will place on service delivery. These include:

- The Public Service Management Act of 1997, which looks at the links between the Department and the Secretary-General, and the Minister and government policy formulation;

- The Freedom of Information Act, 1997, which gives the public full access, subject to some exemptions, to information such as their medical records or the decision-making process used to determine their eligibility for medical cards;

- The continued implementation of the Strategic Management Initiative in the areas of quality customer service, information technology, human resource management and financial management.

This strategy statement also outlines the detailed objectives for each of the divisional areas in the Department, giving a strategic focus to service planning in the system.

CONCLUSION

The current mission statement of the Department of Health is as follows:

> In a partnership with the providers of health care, and in cooperation with other government department, statutory and non-statutory bodies, to protect, promote and restore the wellbeing of the people by ensuring that health and personal social services are planned, managed and delivered to achieve measurable health and social gain and provide the optimum return on resources invested (Department of Health, 1997b).

The mission statement of the Department of Health sums up the current vision or strategic direction aspired to in the health services: "cooperation" rather than "competition", with an emphasis on measurable health and social gain as system targets. If this is to become the guiding force behind the development of health policy and the organisation of services, policy-makers need to have a thorough appreciation of what the situation is at the local level and who are the key stakeholders who should be consulted and involved in the process. While devolvement of decision-making to lower levels is good in principle, it needs to be backed up by a comprehensive communication system to ensure that information and feedback from those at the coal face of service delivery is brought back to those who are funding the service and overseeing its strategic direction. There is a danger that too much emphasis will be put on "forward mapping", the rational approach to planning, and not enough time and emphasis will be given to "backward mapping", the specific behaviours that need to happen at the lowest level of the implementation process. The service planning process is critical to making funding more transparent and for introducing more accountability into the system. How services are funded, planned and organised and the processes of service delivery will need to be understood by all those working in the system. Only then may we aspire to integrated care management of patients that provides the most efficient, effective, high quality and appropriate treatment, in the right environment.

References

Barrington, R. (1987), *Health, Medicine and Politics in Ireland 1900–1970*, Dublin: IPA.

Chubb, B. (1992), *The Government and Politics of Ireland*, 3rd Edition, London: Longman.

Curry, J. (1993), "Chapter 5: Health Services" in *Irish Social Services*, 2nd Edition, Dublin: Institute of Public Administration.

Department of Health (1966), *White Paper: The Health Services and their Future Development*, Dublin: Stationery Office.

Department of Health (1968), "Outline of the Future Hospital System: Report of the Consultative Council on the General Hospital Services", Dublin: Stationery Office.

Department of Health (1984), "Report of the Working Party on the General Medical Services", Dublin: Stationery Office.

Department of Health (1986), "Health: the Wider Dimensions; a Consultative Statement on Health Policy", Dublin: Stationery Office.

Department of Health (1989), "Report of the Commission on Health Funding", Dublin: Stationery Office.

Department of Health (1990), "Community Medicine and Public Health — the Future", Report of a Working Party, Dublin: Stationery Office.

Department of Health (1991), Reports (three) of the Dublin Hospital Initiative Group, 1990–1991, Dublin: Stationery Office.

Department of Health, Comhairle na nOspideal, Postgraduate Medical and Dental Board (1993), "Medical Manpower in Acute Hospitals, A Discussion Document", March.

Department of Health (1994), "Shaping a Healthier Future: A Strategy for Effective Health Care in the 1990s", Dublin: Stationery Office

Department of Health (1995), "Report of the Expert Group on the Blood Transfusion Service Board", Dublin: Stationery Office.

Department of Health (1997a), "Interim Report of the Task Force on the Eastern Regional Health Authority", June, Dublin: Stationery Office.

Department of Health (1997b), "Statement of Strategy", Dublin: Stationery Office.

Department of Health (1997c), "Enhancing the Partnership: Report of the Working Groups on the Implementation of the Health Strategy in relation to persons with a Mental Handicap", Dublin: Stationery Office.

Department of Health (1998), "Strategy Statement 1998–2001: Working for Health and Well-Being", Dublin: Stationery Office.

Dooney, S. and J. O'Toole (1992), "Chapter 9: The Health Service" in *Irish Government Today*, Dublin: Gill and Macmillan.

Hensey, B. (1988), *The Health Services of Ireland*, 4th Edition, Dublin: IPA.

Institute of Public Administration (various years), Fact Sheets on Various Aspects of the Irish Health Service, Health Resource Centre, Dublin: IPA.

McKevitt, D. (1990), *Health Care Policy in Ireland: A Study in Control*, Cork: Hibernian University Press.

National Economic and Social Council (1987), "Community Care Services: an Overview", Dublin: NESC.

Robins, J. (1997), *Reflections on Health: Commemorating Fifty Years of the Department of Health, 1947–1997*, Dublin: Department of Health.

2

REFLECTIONS ON FUTURE STRUCTURES IN THE HEALTH SERVICES

Jerry O'Dwyer

INTRODUCTION

The formal structures for the planning, delivery and evaluation of the health services in Ireland remained unchanged in the 25 years between 1970 and 1995. Changes are now, however, beginning to take place, primarily in response to the Health Strategy published in 1994. If there is anything of which we can be reasonably certain in the rapidly changing world of the health services, it is that future structures will follow strategy.

It is possible to identify a number of factors which must be taken into account by those responsible for ensuring that structures support effectiveness and efficiency. The structures must be designed primarily to achieve the health gain and social gain targets, which will be set out in strategies at regular intervals. They must be as simple as possible, sensible to those who operate them and easily understood by those who must access them. To support change and complexity, they need to be flexible and allow for a great deal of informal working, which characterises many Irish organisations and is particularly suited to current and prospective organisational needs.

Future structures must, at all levels, support a high degree of accountability and transparency. They must support a high level of responsiveness to the needs and expectations of the patient and facilitate greater involvement of the community, particularly groups promoting health or supporting patients with chronic diseases, in contributing to policy formulation and evaluation. They must support and encourage far greater involvement of clinical staff in policy formulation and review and, in particular, the management of services at the point of delivery. The increasing need to work with other agencies in order to achieve health gain and social gain must be reflected at national, regional and local levels. Perhaps most importantly for the long-term wellbeing of the system, the structures must facilitate accurate and sensitive identification of needs, development of programmes to meet those needs, and the objective measurement of their impact.

THE CHANGING CONTEXT

In suggesting how future structures may develop, it is necessary to make a number of assumptions with regard to the context in which they are likely to operate. It is assumed that the public health system will continue to be centrally funded from taxation. The relative success of Ireland in controlling overall expenditure, in setting and achieving national priorities, and the desire to ensure equity across the whole country and between groups with different needs all point to a continuation of the present system.

It is also assumed that significant and increasing income will continue to remain available to health boards and hospitals from the treatment of private patients covered by health insurance. The extent to which a separate private system will develop, whether in the provision of hospital- or community-based services, will depend on the success of the public services in meeting identifiable shortcomings, particularly in the next three to five years when the economy is likely to remain vibrant.

It is reasonable to assume that changes in structures will not be driven by any particular ideology and that the market model will not be adopted. It is much more likely that changes in structures will be evolutionary, based on experience and evidence, responding to an agenda which is primarily dominated by the requirements of health strategy, formulated in accordance with overall government policies. Nevertheless, it is likely that there will be a willingness, in relation to parts of the system that are not performing, to demolish existing structures and to substitute something more appropriate.

It is further assumed that health boards will remain at the centre of the delivery system. Although it would facilitate integration, it seems unlikely that there will be a move to multi-competent authorities at regional level and this will require that health boards demonstrate enthusiasm and ability in developing effective inter-agency working.

The overall system is likely to be much more responsive to external influences. These will include developments in the European Union, in North/South co-operation, and in the development of increasingly more reliable international indicators of health and health service performance. The health promotion, prevention and public health aspects of the system are likely to receive greater prominence and will, in certain respects, have to be strengthened. For example, the growth of infections, food-borne and blood-borne diseases, the threats arising from the abuse and overuse of antibiotics, and the implications of the rapid development of bioethics and genetics will all have to be reflected in the structures of health agencies and the expertise required in the broad area of public health.

Quality assurance will have to be built into all structures and systems. This is likely to see the emergence of further regulation; the development, perhaps on a voluntary basis initially, of various forms of accreditation; and the development of more contractual-type relationships between professionals and those to whom they provide advice, treatment or care.

The interface between the various sectors of care is undergoing continuous change and that change may be more marked in the future. In particular, it is probable that the general practice/specialist practice interface will come under increasing pressure. It is probable that patients with acute conditions, requiring specialist medical or surgical intervention, will seek to bypass general practice and go directly to the specialist whom they consider can best deal with their condition. Those with more chronic conditions may be more demanding of their general practitioner, if the latter is to remain the gatekeeper, guaranteeing continuity and co-ordination of care. Such continuity may be less highly regarded by the patient than by the professional, depending on the condition. In this, there is a challenge to the role of the general practitioner.

These are some of the considerations that may influence the future development of structures throughout the health system in Ireland. Against this background, the changes and developments which are likely to emerge in the principal agencies are now considered.

DEPARTMENT OF HEALTH AND CHILDREN

The change in the title of the Department in June 1997, to give it enhanced responsibilities in relation to children, is of considerable significance. It places on the Department a responsibility to develop, monitor and review (on behalf of the Government) an overall strategy in relation to children. In addition, it gives it a lead responsibility in ensuring the health and wellbeing of children at risk and proposing solutions to some of the more intractable social problems. These include the care of children who are out of the control of their parents or guardians and the development of services for children whose lives are blighted by social and economic disadvantage. Structures must be evolved to gain cross-departmental agreement on an overall strategy, to ensure the implementation of the changes that it will require, and monitoring of the effectiveness with which the strategy is being implemented. This is one of the more demanding cross-departmental tasks assigned to any Department and will require the development and implementation of much better processes than have heretofore been available to the Department to influence the policies and practices of other Departments.

This may be the most obvious challenge to the Department but it is certainly not the only one. In common with other Departments, it must now be geared to support the Minister in discharging a very high level of accountability to the Dáil, and to his or her colleagues in Government. The greater specificity in the programme of incoming Governments, and the requirement under the Public Service Management Act, 1997, to publish a strategy statement for the Department and lay it before the Houses of the Oireachtas, provide a template against which each Minister will be judged in his or her stewardship of the Department. The Department is now subject to much greater accountability to the Dáil through the various reports of the Comptroller and Auditor General and the strengthened Dáil committee system.

The structures within the Department must reflect these realities. They must also reflect the need to produce good overall strategic plans for the system, and demonstrate an ability to co-ordinate their implementation and evaluate their impact. The focus will increasingly be on the measurement and improvement of outcomes, on the reduction of premature deaths and on the development of better prevention, care and rehabilitation policies for various target groups, e.g. children, the elderly, women, the disabled and the mentally handicapped. While dealing with these issues, the Department must continue to ensure that the overall system is well managed, that its structures and systems are effective and efficient and that it is held accountable for the use of the resources which it is allocated on an annual or multi-annual basis.

The framework for the health boards' accountability to the Minister, through the Department, is set out in the Health (Amendment) (No. 3) Act, 1996. It is, by far, the most specific piece of accountability legislation currently affecting the Irish public service and it requires, inter alia, the production of an annual service plan by each health board, within the limits of the resources available to it. This now forms the primary basis of each health board's interaction with the Department. It is very likely that, in the near future, the Department will have to change its structure to reflect the importance of this relationship and to facilitate quicker and more efficient processing and monitoring of service plans. The challenge in any such restructuring is to ensure that those involved in overseeing the work of the agencies and those who are mainly involved in policy formulation and review remain close to each other and work co-operatively on the basis of shared intelligence and analysis. The Department's consciousness of the agencies as customers, who must be supported in the discharge of their difficult task, reflects a wider change in thinking throughout the public service which will continue to influence the design of structures and systems.

The Department's responsibilities in relation to children, to food safety, to health promotion and disease prevention, to the reduction in the incidence of cardiovascular disease, cancer and accidents and to the reduction in the demand for drugs, all require that its structures facilitate very close co-operation and efficient working arrangements with a range of other Departments. It is not possible to design a neat structure, such as one dedicated unit, to handle this very wide range of contacts. The main requirement is to see other Departments as essential partners in achieving improvements for the good of the whole community. As more experience is gained of cross-departmental working, it is possible that it will demand less time from very senior staff, but new areas of co-operation must always be led by officers who are seen to carry the full authority of the Minister and the Department in achieving the agreed objectives.

The Department must also make decisions on how it should be structured to give the necessary impetus to developing services to provide for the needs of the old and the very old. This is likely to require the development of a project group, drawing on most areas of the Department and led by a senior officer who will work closely with the Minister or Minister of State responsible for the sector. This is one example of the type of work that has led to the development of increased expertise in the management of multidisciplinary and multi-interest project teams. Many officers in the Department must in future cope with three types of responsibility: a corporate responsibility for the overall work of the organisation; a direct responsibility for a particular sector or function; and a team responsibility for a project or a number of projects that cut across formal organisation structures.

There are three other areas worthy of mention in considering the likely changes of structures within the Department. First of all, the Chief Medical Officer and staff are faced with considerable challenges in developing appropriate policies and practices in the fields of bioethics and genetics. These are both rapidly developing areas and, as yet, full policy frameworks and legislation have not been put in place. The second area is coming to terms with the health impact of various aspects of the environment. A policy paper on this is likely to be published before the end of this year and it is very likely that some structural changes, to enhance its ability to work better with various other departments and agencies in this field, will be required.

Finally, one can reasonably anticipate that the international dimension of the Department's work will grow significantly in the years ahead. The public health framework likely to be put in place from 2000 onwards under the Amsterdam Treaty will place a considerable burden on member states to contribute to potentially powerful data banks on various aspects of health and health services; to help develop networks throughout the Union which will seek to identify and spread best practice; and to cope, perhaps through the provision of bilateral or multilateral assistance, with the advent of up to ten new applicant countries in the first decade of the next century.

In summary, the Department will continue to devolve such remaining executive work as it now retains to the proposed new Eastern Regional Health Authority and to Health Boards; it will reshape its structures to deal more smoothly and efficiently with the health boards and the other parts of the delivery system; it will devote more time and energy to cross-departmental working without greatly changing its structures; and it will strengthen its ability to formulate policy and evaluate impact, primarily by concentrating on the needs of care groups and on the reduction of the prime causes of premature death.

HEALTH BOARDS

The role and responsibilities of health boards and their Chief Executive Officers have been clearly delineated in the Health (Amendment) (No. 3) Act, 1996. The governance role of the board, although not expressed in such terms, has been emphasised. The clear line drawn between governance and management is one that has been well accepted in the health services for many years but has not previously been so clearly defined. The membership of health boards, drawn from public representatives, persons elected by the professions and persons appointed by the Minister, is unlikely to change in the foreseeable future. However, it is possible that changes proposed in relation to local authorities may, in due course, have some effect on the way in which the public representatives are appointed to the boards.

The boards, with the advice and support of their managements, have the task of identifying the priority needs in their area and measuring the impact of the services which they provide. Needs assessment, at present, is primarily a matter for professionals, often based on their contacts with various representative groups. It is likely, however, that future assessment of needs and measurement of satisfaction with services will be more influenced by the views of the population within each board's catchment area. This will involve the development of various survey techniques, wider and more frequent consultation, the use of focus groups and more objective measurement of patients' degree of satisfaction with the services they receive.

Health boards now have considerable experience of managing services across a wide range of programmes. They have taken steps in recent times to review their structures. This review is likely to lead to a division at top management level between those responsible for the operational aspects of services and those who are responsible for the overall health needs of the population that the board serves. More particularly, the boards are now faced with the challenge of developing structures, systems and expertise to contract formally with voluntary hospitals, with agencies providing services for the mentally handicapped and with other large voluntary organisations for the provision of services.

Much of the emphasis up to now has been on the amount of input which the health board would provide. There has been less emphasis on the output and the quality of care to be provided as part of the contracted service. While this change of emphasis will mainly affect the proposed Eastern Regional Health Authority, it will have some impact on all health boards. It is likely that all boards will initially rely heavily on the experience now being gained in the arrangements which have been agreed with certain agencies providing services for the mentally handicapped under the Mid-Western and Southern Health Boards.

The managements of health boards have recognised for quite some time the need to work together to handle a range of executive work now associated with the Department, to maximise their purchasing and negotiating power and to provide a more co-ordinated delivery of services. It is now likely that an agency to facilitate this formally and take on a very wide range of responsibilities will be established within the next year. This will service the needs of both the boards and the Department, insofar as it will facilitate the completion of the devolution programme drawn up by the Department. Health Boards must also develop structures and systems for closer and more extensive working with local authorities, with the Departments of Education and Justice, and with the Garda. They must also work closely with a variety of agencies, including the Department of Social, Community and Family Affairs, with which it already has arrangements for the delivery of a number of services such as supplementary welfare payments.

When the agency to facilitate boards to perform a range of functions on a joint basis is established, it will create the conditions under which the boards collectively can form a more direct relationship with the European Commission. It will, of course, be necessary to agree the functions which the board collectively should perform in this area, as distinct from those to be performed by the Department.

There is little doubt that all boards will become much more conscious of health in the EU context over the next decade.

Health board structures will, at local level, have to respond to their increasing responsibilities in relation to children, particularly children at risk. There will also be an increasing requirement to promote healthy behaviour among all sectors of the population, to work with a variety of agencies in combating social disadvantage and poverty, and to ensure the highest possible standards of safety in relation to food, water and air. At a functional level, it is probable that all health boards will have to reassess their structure and competencies in attracting and retaining suitable staff. In a growing economy, with a reducing number of eighteen-year-olds and an increase in the numbers of elderly people, health boards will face increasing difficulties in attracting and retaining suitably qualified and experienced staff. This is already evident in relation to certain categories of nursing and paramedical staff and we can see, from the experiences of other countries, the challenges we face. It is, therefore, likely that responsibility for recruitment will shift from the Local Appointments Commission to the health boards. Future modes of recruitment and the forms of employment by health boards will reflect the reality of a scarcity of suitable staff.

ACUTE HOSPITALS

Acute hospitals will continue to be subject to more extensive and rapid change than any other part of the health system. More resources will have to be invested in their management. The management structures in major voluntary hospitals and in major acute hospitals under health boards are likely to develop along similar lines.

Steps are already being taken to delineate more clearly the governance and management functions within the large hospitals. Both functions are still relatively underdeveloped. Whereas considerable attention has been given to the strengthening of management in recent years, the responsibilities of governance have not been subject to the same degree of consideration and development. Members of hospital boards are non-executive directors of complex organisations dealing with some of the most difficult ethical, legal and quality issues. The demands made on people filling these roles and, in particular, the demands on the chairperson, are likely to be reflected in the means through which the members are selected and supported during the term of their membership.

The role of the chief executive of the hospital and the management team will continue to change. Their authority in relation to operational matters is likely to be strengthened. Their accountability will increase accordingly and will become more transparent. They are likely to devote more of their energy to creating an environment in which various professions with clinical responsibility can play a greater role in managing the day-to-day work of the hospital. That environment is likely to be significantly determined by an overall strategy for the hospital, which will have to be produced, in the first instance, by the chief executive of the hospital. Within the management team, the scope of the patient services task is likely to be extended significantly to reflect much greater concern with quality assurance and patient satisfaction. Human resources, systems and risk management are other areas which will go through a period of sustained development over the next decade and which will remain critical to the hospital's ability to achieve its agreed objectives.

The management team of a large hospital will, in practice, have dual accountability. Its primary accountability will be to its own board, but it will also be the group through which the hospital discharges its accountability to the local health board. It is likely that the contract agreements between a health board and the major hospital will place responsibilities on the hospital, not only in relation to the provision of services but also in relation to co-operation with other sectors of the health services, in the interest of efficiency and co-ordination. It is probable, for example, that the nature and extent of the services to be provided to general practitioners will be more clearly defined. The arrangements for rehabilitation and for transfer to other services, following the acute phase of care, will be pre-planned with greater rigour and on a normative basis. The hospital will also have a large role to play in co-operating with the health board in measuring outcomes.

Steps are already being taken, through a number of pilot programmes, to facilitate greater clinical involvement by doctors, nurses and paramedicals in the operational management of the large acute hospitals. It is probable that most hospitals will adopt structures based on clinical directorates, but there is still a great deal of scope for experimentation and development with regard to the processes which best suit any particular hospital. In parallel with the greater responsibility for operational matters, the clinicians will also play a greater role in the evaluation of the work done and in the formulation of policy. The development of strategic statements by hospitals on a regular basis should greatly facilitate the involvement of a far greater proportion of staff in shaping the hospitals' objectives and in acquiring a sense of ownership with regard to their achievement.

It is also probable that hospitals will adopt an appropriate form of disease management programme for the major conditions which they treat and for chronic conditions. This should, in turn, necessitate a closer linkage of medicine and surgery and relevant support services, and the development of cross-functional teams. It is also likely to encourage identification of needs through working with patients and their representatives, with greater emphasis on pharmacological compliance, self care, and the tracking of outcomes by linking data from diagnostic related groups with data on medication usage.

The steps that are already being taken to link smaller hospitals more closely with large acute hospitals are likely to continue. The acute hospital services will be characterised by clusters of closely related hospitals which complement each other and facilitate the free movement of staff and patients to achieve the best use of resources and to provide a high quality service to all patients. It is likely, for example, that such clusters will form the basis of employment of non-consultant hospital doctors in the early years of their career. Such clustering may also facilitate the development of better generalist and specialist training and so help to address the current medical manpower problems.

Major hospitals will, therefore, be more outward-looking in their orientation, be more concerned with co-ordination with other hospitals and with other sectors within the health system. This will be reflected in the structures through which the hospital is managed. It is likely, for example, that the typical chief executive of a major acute hospital will spend a high proportion of his or her time negotiating on behalf of the hospital with various external agencies. This will create the need for a deputy who will take responsibility for the day-to-day operations of the hospital. The chief executive and members of the management team are also likely to be invited to participate in various policy reviews and in project teams which range in their work across a number of agencies. The structures to accommodate these developments that are likely to evolve are unlikely to be prescribed by the Department or health board, and will probably remain part of the informal rather than the formal structures through which services are planned and delivered.

SPECIALIST AGENCIES

In addition to health boards, a number of specialist agencies will continue to report directly to the Department. These include the Blood Transfusion Services Board, the Irish Medicines Board, Comhairle na nOspidéal, the Food Safety Authority of Ireland and the Post Graduate Medical and Dental Board. At present, the Voluntary Health Insurance Board is wholly owned by the Minister for Health, to whom it is accountable, but it is likely that there will be a change in the status and the reporting relationship of the Board in the near future. This is particularly likely given EU requirements in relation to the provision of private health insurance and the conflict between the regulatory function of the Minister and his or her ownership of VHI.

It is not anticipated that the number of specialist agencies will increase to any significant extent in the foreseeable future. The Department is committed to a regular review of the role and functioning of each of these specialist agencies. At the present time, the Irish Medicines Board and the Blood Transfusion Service Board are the subject of extensive restructuring and strengthening. The Food Safety Authority is being established through a new Act. The role and the functioning of Comhairle na nOspidéal and the Post Graduate Medical and Dental Board will, no doubt, be the subject of some consideration in the context of a wide-ranging review of future medical manpower policy.

The challenge to all of these bodies is to remain relevant to the task to be performed, to achieve a high level of fitness in their governance and management, and to be accountable to the Minister in relation to outcomes and efficiency. As in the case of acute hospitals, it is likely that there will be greater emphasis on the governance function. In certain bodies, notably the Food Safety Authority, The Blood Transfusion Service Board and the Irish Medicines Board, there will be a sustained high level of concern with ensuring the safety of product made available to the consumer. This will, in turn, require the development of high level expertise in gathering and analysing intelligence from here and from other countries, learning to balance the duty of care with very low level or potentially negligible risks, and retaining the confidence of the Government of the day and the public in the information and commentary which it makes available. It is likely, therefore, that internal structures within these organisations will necessarily change on a regular basis and that new types of expertise will have to be acquired, on either a staff or contract basis.

PROFESSIONAL REGULATORY BODIES

The bodies regulating the professions of medicine, nursing, pharmacy and opticians all operate under statute. Each of them is, at this stage, seeking a review of the relevant legislation and it is likely that this will materialise over the next few years. The basic principle of self-regulation is likely to remain unchallenged but, reflecting development in the wider society, the bodies are likely to be required to conduct their business on a more transparent basis and to give greater representation to the consumer interest. It is also likely that, following extensive consultation that has taken place for a number of years, legislation will be enacted which will regulate a number of the paramedical professions, including physiotherapy, occupational therapy and social work. Consideration will also have to be given to the regulation of various forms of counselling, although this is likely to be at least as difficult and contentious as reaching agreement with the paramedical professions.

TRADE UNIONS AND PATIENT ORGANISATIONS

Successive Governments have been committed, with the Irish Congress of Trade Unions and the employers' organisations, to planning and managing many aspects of our society on a partnership basis. Depending on the success of Partnership 2000, it is reasonable to assume that the commitment to partnership will continue and that the structures to which partnership is made to work will be developed and strengthened over the coming years. The Health Service Employers Agency has brought together all of the major employers within the health services. It has a much wider remit than the maintenance of good industrial relations and the capacity which has been built into its structures in relation to change management should, with co-operation from employers and trade unions, facilitate the development of real partnership. Such a development, will, undoubtedly, require changes on both the management and union side, not least to ensure the transmission right down through the respective organisations of the principles, commitments and practices which are agreed from time to time at the top level. While there are models in other countries which can be helpful to us in developing the practice of partnership, we will have to develop our own solutions in many instances and it is unlikely that all of these solutions will work well from the beginning.

A somewhat different form of partnership is likely to develop with organisations representing patients. We are now very familiar and well practised in dealing with organisations which represent groups with chronic conditions. Many of these are well established, highly organised and well co-ordinated. Their mission is generally clear and they represent the interest of groups of people over a very long period. In the case of patients with acute conditions, their interest tends to be more ephemeral. It is more difficult for people who wish to represent acute hospital patients to develop an organisation which is representative and serves the needs of patients. While this is an area in which developments can be expected, it is quite difficult to envisage the forms of organisation and representation that are likely to prove effective and acceptable. Nevertheless, all entities within the health services must be better geared to provide a truly patient-centred service, to respond positively to suggestions, to learn from complaints and to be at least as much concerned with service as any retail organisation whose survival depends on the quality of what it offers, the consistency of its response and the reputation which it develops.

CONCLUSIONS

The mission statement of the Department of Health and Children, quoted at the end of Chapter 1, emphasises the achievement of real health and social gain through co-operation with many statutory and non-statutory bodies. It also highlights the importance of achieving value for money in the use of resources.

That mission statement is unlikely to change significantly in the foreseeable future. The structures through which the overall health system is planned, delivered, evaluated and made sensible to the people who use it must always be seen to be promoting the achievement of that mission. The strategies that will be developed from time to time to support the implementation of the mission must be the main determinants of the structure. The extent of change in the structure will, therefore, be determined by the nature and extent of the changes which are reflected in these strategies.

References

"Action Programme for the Millennium", Programme of the Fianna Fáil/ Progressive Democrat Government, June 1997.

Department of Health (1994), "Shaping a Healthier Future — A Strategy of Effective Health Care in the 1990s", Dublin: Stationery Office.

Department of Health and Children (1998), "Working for Health and Wellbeing", Strategy statement 1998–2001, Dublin: Stationery Office, April.

Kings Fund (1998), *The Quest for Excellence — What is Good Health Care?* London: Kings Fund Publishing.

Robins, Joe (ed.) (1997), *Reflections on Health: Commemorating Fifty Years of the Department of Health 1947–1997*, Dublin: Institute of Public Administration.

US Health Care Advisory Board (1997), "Planning and Implementing Disease Management Programmes", Review article published by US Health Care Advisory Board, August.

3

"A Particular Problem in the East . . ."[1]

Donal O'Shea

Introduction

On 27 November 1996, the then Minister for Health, Mr Michael Noonan TD, announced that the government had agreed to his proposals

> . . . for the establishment of an Eastern Regional Health Authority which would have responsibility for the funding of all health and personal social services in Dublin, Kildare and Wicklow. Under the new arrangements, all services, both voluntary and statutory, will be funded by the new Authority, facilitating more integrated planning, delivery and evaluation of health and personal social services in the area. I believe this will enable the Authority to promote a more effective, efficient and patient/consumer friendly delivery system in the region.

The Minister also announced his intention to set up a "high level Task Force to oversee and manage the implementation of his proposals". The first full meeting of this Task Force took place in February 1997.

The announcement outlined some key elements of the Government's decisions:

- It was being taken in response to the 1994 Health Strategy *Shaping a Healthier Future* and the "particular problem in the Eastern Health Board area", identified in Chapter Three of that document;

---

[1] *Shaping a Healthier Future*, p. 32.

- The new Eastern Regional Health Authority will replace the Eastern Health Board and will be responsible for the funding of all health and personal social services, both statutory and voluntary, in Counties Dublin, Kildare and Wicklow;

- Public representatives will hold the majority on the new Authority. Councillors will be nominated to the Authority by Dublin Corporation and the County Councils of Fingal, South Dublin, Dun Laoghaire-Rathdown, Kildare and Wicklow;

- The Authority will also include persons drawn from the voluntary hospitals, mental handicap agencies and other voluntary bodies;

- The Authority will be managed through three Area Health Councils whose members will be drawn from the membership of the Authority;

- Area Managers, reporting to the Chief Executive Officer, will be appointed to correspond with the Area Health Councils;

- The proposed boundaries of the three areas were set out into Northern, South Western and South Eastern Areas.

It was envisaged that the full transition to the new arrangements would take two to three years.

THE HISTORY

The hospital services in the Eastern region have a long and interesting history. Many of the current voluntary hospitals date back to the early 1700s. For example, the Charitable Infirmary, or Jervis St Hospital, since transferred as part of the new Beaumont Hospital, dates from 1718. Mercers Hospital opened as a ten-bed institution in 1724. Dr Steevens Hospital accepted its first patient in 1733. The Rotunda Hospital was established as the first "lying-in hospital" in 1745 and was financed by concerts and entertainments.

The Hospital for Incurables, now the Royal Hospital Donnybrook, began in a few rooms in Fleet Street in 1743 under the patronage of members of the Charitable Musical Society of Crow Street.

The Adelaide Hospital has provided a focus for Protestant participation in the Irish health services since its foundation in Bride Street in 1839. The Adelaide Institution and Protestant Hospital reopened in Peter Street in 1858 as the Adelaide Hospital and has now moved to the Tallaght site as part of the new Adelaide and Meath Hospital incorporating the National Children's Hospital.

The Meath Hospital was established in 1753 in the Coombe district and moved five times before settling in Heytesbury Street in 1822. Its first treasurer was one Arthur Guinness, who achieved even greater fame in other fields. It has also now moved to Tallaght as part of the new hospital.

During the 19th century, other well-known hospitals were established. These include the Coombe Hospital 1823, originally intended as a general hospital but becoming the Coombe Lying-in Hospital in 1825.

St Vincent's Hospital opened for the sick poor in 1834 on the site of the Earl of Meath's Georgian mansion on St Stephens Green, transferring to Elm Park in 1970. In 1851, the Congregation of the Sisters of Mercy purchased a fifteen-acre site in Eccles Street on which the Mater Misericordiae Hospital still stands, its magnificent building designed by Francis Johnston, and the great front on Eccles Street by John Bourke.

The longest lineage of the current Dublin hospitals is arguably that of St James's Hospital, which can trace its ancestry back nearly three centuries to a 1703 Act of the Irish Parliament which established a workhouse in James's Street.

The history of public health services in the region is equally long and varied. The earliest legislation dates back to 1703 with the setting up of workhouses; county infirmaries date from 1765; public health services from 1878 with the appointment of dispensary doctors; county medical officers from 1925. The services over the centuries were administered variously by Poor Law Commissioners, Boards of Guardians and then the Local Authorities. The Eastern Health Board was set up in 1970 as the direct successor for health services of the Dublin Health Authority and the Wicklow and Kildare County Councils.

Over the past decade or so, there have been a number of studies by committees and working groups which have addressed the structural problems of the Eastern region. These include:

- *Health: the Wider Dimensions* (1986)

- The Commission on Health Funding (1989)

- The Hospital Efficiency Review Group (1990)

- The Dublin Hospital Initiative Group (1990)

- *Shaping a Healthier Future* or the National Health Strategy (1994).

The core problem identified by these successive reports could be summarised as:

a) The absence of a single authority with responsibility for planning, delivery and co-ordination of services for the region;

b) Over-centralised decision-making within the health board and the lack of an appropriate management structure at district level, given the increase in the population over the last 25 years;

c) The need for better communication and co-operation between the voluntary sector and the health board.

THE ISSUES

While recognising the undoubted strengths of our health system, the Health Strategy identified a number of weaknesses which had to be resolved, including:

- Lack of sufficiently focused goals or targets;

- Lack of information to support these goals;

- Insufficient attention to tackling the main causes of premature mortality (life expectancy here is lower than the EU average);

- Waiting times too long;

- Inadequate linkages between complementary services such as hospitals, general practitioners and other community services;

- Community-based services not complementary nor substitutive for institutional care;

- Organisational and management structures out of date.

The main elements of the Health Strategy — including the pursuit of the concepts of health gain and social gain; the planning of services based on measured needs; the principle of equity, including equity of access; improved efficiency and accountability — are set out in a context which relies on improvements in the framework within which services are planned, funded, monitored and evaluated. They call for a network that supports improved linkages, both vertical and horizontal, within and between the services to facilitate co-operation, collaboration, holism and comprehensiveness.

The document finds that, while deficiencies apply to the structure as a whole:

> . . . there is a particular problem in the Eastern Health Board area. Here to a greater extent than elsewhere significant services are provided by voluntary agencies, but there is no single authority with an overall responsibility to co-ordinate all services and to ensure appropriate linkages between them.
>
> Because of the need to have a body with comprehensive responsibility for all health and personal social services in the Eastern region, there will be a new health authority to replace the Eastern Health Board.

The population of the eight health regions is shown in Table 3.1. In 1971, the population of the Eastern Health Board region was 990,491. By 1996, this had risen to 1,293,964 an increase of 303,473 or 31 per cent.

This increase is equal to the current total population of the North Eastern Health Board region and is much greater than that of either the Midlands or North-West. Despite this very significant growth, the Eastern Health Board has remained a very centralised body, in many ways even more centralised than Boards serving significantly smaller populations.

Table 3.1: Population of Health Board Areas

Region	Census 1996
Midland	205,252
North-Western	210,112
North-Eastern	305,703
Mid-Western	316,875
Western	351,875
South-Eastern	390,946
Southern	546,209
Eastern	1,293,964

In addressing this issue, the Health Strategy states:

> In view of the size of the population to be served and the range and complexity of the services to be provided, the new authority will operate through a number of management areas within the region. The emphasis at area level will be to achieve the maximum integration of hospital and community services and to reflect local needs and priorities.

At present, the Eastern Health Board is statutorily responsible for services in Counties Dublin, Kildare and Wicklow. However, in practice, the bulk of the general hospital services and much of the mental handicap provision in the region are funded directly by the Department of Health and Children and do not have any statutory links with the Board.

The Eastern Health Board employs approximately 9,000 staff and has a direct budget of £475 million from the Department of Health and Children (See Figures 3.1 and 3.2). The Board delivers a wide range of services including environmental health services; dental services; AIDS/HIV/drug abuse services; child care and family support services; services for the elderly; services for people with physical and sensory disabilities; services for the homeless; community health services; counselling services; mental health services; public health services; medical services; some general hospital services; and some mental handicap services.

Figure 3.1: 1998 Funding, Eastern Region (£1.3 billion)

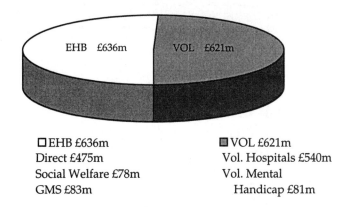

☐ EHB £636m
Direct £475m
Social Welfare £78m
GMS £83m

☒ VOL £621m
Vol. Hospitals £540m
Vol. Mental
    Handicap £81m

Figure 3.2: Staffing Numbers, Eastern Region

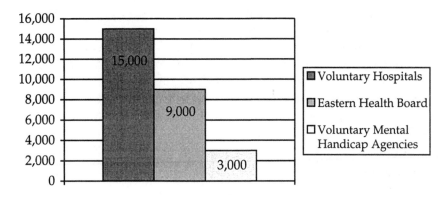

In addition to providing its own services, the Eastern Health Board also funds some voluntary providers directly, including approximately 300 small voluntary groups and associations (Committees for the Elderly, Community Playgroups, Youth Development Groups, etc). This funding accounts for some £70 million of the Board's budget. The Board also provides the GMS service (£83 million) and a range of services funded by the Department of Social, Community and Family Affairs (£78 million).

The Department of Health and Children provides direct funding of £540 million to 29 voluntary hospitals and agencies in the Eastern region. Together these employ over 15,000 people. The Department

also provides direct funding of over £81 million to the six largest
voluntary mental handicap organisations, whose headquarters are
located in the Eastern region. These organisations employ over 3,000
staff.

The total funding for health and personal social services in the
Eastern region amounts to £1.3 billion and total employment is of the
order of 27,000 staff.

The functions of the health authority in each region are set out in
the Health Strategy as follows:

- Deciding on a multi-annual strategic plan based on the identified
  needs of its population and taking account of statutory requirements and national policy guidelines;

- Determining, at the beginning of each year, the level of services
  to be provided within the expenditure limits set by the allocation;

- Agreeing and submitting to the Minister a budget for those services within the expenditure limits determined by the allocation.

The current Eastern Health Board, being effectively responsible for
funding and co-ordinating only half of the services in the Eastern region, cannot effectively carry out this role.

THE PROCESS

Within the framework and parameters announced by the Minister in
November 1996 and on the basis of the Health Strategy, the Task
Force set about its work of formulating proposals to Government as
requested. An extensive consultation process was begun with all interested parties. Contact was made with all providers, both statutory
and voluntary, within the Eastern region, to invite submissions.
Similar invitations were sent to the main staff associations, the universities, other third level institutions and private hospitals. Meetings
and discussions were held with many of the principal parties involved, including the members of the Board and management of the
Eastern Health Board, management and owners of voluntary hospi-

tals, voluntary agencies and organisations providing services to persons with a mental handicap, and some staff associations.

On 30 June 1997, a report outlining the proposed structure for a new Authority, its Area Councils and its relationships with all providers, both statutory and voluntary, was presented to the Minister for Health and Children, Brian Cowen TD. The report also dealt with Authority and Area Councils memberships, the boundaries of the Areas, the setting up of district units of membership and issues of accountability. It set out the main objectives of the new arrangements with a clear focus on an improved service to patients and clients.

Before the end of July, the Minister announced the Government's acceptance of the report as the basis for legislation and ordered the publication of the report. The report itself became the focus for continuing consultation with all of the main parties outlined above, the results of which were available to those involved in formulating the proposals for legislation.

It is expected that the Bill setting up the new Authority will be before the Houses of the Oireachtas during the last quarter of 1998.

In the meantime, the Task Force has continued its work of setting up the arrangements for the functioning of the new Authority. Staffs from the voluntary hospitals, the voluntary mental handicap agencies, the Eastern Health Board and the Department of Health and Children are working with the Task Force on strategy committees and working groups to put these arrangements in place.

The timetable is ultimately a matter for Government and the legislators, but the Task Force is working to a target of being ready for A-day (Authority-day) by 1 January 1999 or any day afterwards.

THE PROPOSALS

The Minister's proposal of November 1996 stated that the new Authority would:

- Replace the Eastern Health Board;
- Take on the function of funding of the voluntary providers in the region currently carried out by the Department of Health;

- Assume responsibility for the co-ordination and integration of all health and personal social services in the region;

- Be managed through three Area Health Councils.

It is now envisaged that the role of the new Authority at central level would be:

- Identifying the health and social needs of the population in its region;

- Procuring funding from the Minister for Health for services in the region;

- Planning the services in the region, including setting outcomes targets to meet identified needs;

- Commissioning, by means of service agreements with various providers, measures or services to achieve agreed objectives;

- Allocating resources to each of the providers, statutory and voluntary;

- Working with other agencies within and outside the region to protect and promote health;

- Monitoring and reviewing the services in the region against targets.

The Authority would determine overall policy in relation to health and social services in the region, taking into account national policy and the needs and requirements of the Region and its Areas. It would inherit responsibility for the very wide range of services currently provided by the Eastern Health Board, mainly in the community health, continuing care and personal social services fields.

During the consultation process, very strong concerns were expressed regarding a conflict of interest which might arise if the same body, whether the board of the central Authority or an Area Health Council, were responsible both for funding some services (i.e. in the voluntary sector) and directly providing others (i.e. those currently provided by the Eastern Health Board).

It is now envisaged that the Authority at central level should have no management role in direct delivery of services. Services currently provided by the Eastern Health Board should be provided by the three Area Councils, with significant responsibility being legally vested in them for that purposes. This would then create a simple structure in which the Central Authority would have, in effect, similar arrangement with all its providers — the 35 voluntary agencies and the three area councils.

There would be no change in the status or operational autonomy of any voluntary provider. Their ownership would not change, their governing bodies (whether boards of management or trustees) would remain and would retain all of their functions, and there would be no change in the existing personnel and recruitment arrangements. The close co-operation between the universities and their associated hospitals would be maintained. What would change is that voluntary providers in the Eastern Region would receive their funding from the Eastern Regional Health Authority, instead of from the Department of Health, by means of an agreement between each voluntary provider and the Authority.

These arrangements between the Authority and its providers would be formalised and would be by way of individual provider agreements and provider plans. Provider agreements covering provision of three to five years would set out general parameters as to the nature and quantum of services to be provided. A more detailed formal agreement, the provider plan, would be drawn in the context of the provider agreement but would be far more detailed and would reflect the level of funding for the year. The elements of this provider plan would include:

- Quantum of service to be provided
- Effectiveness
- Efficiency
- Equity
- Quality
- Access

- Appropriateness of care

- Responsiveness to the public.

Both agreements and plans would include a requirement for the supply of the information required to enable the Authority carry out its function of monitoring and evaluation of the service provision.

There would also be a provision for Providers' Forums in which the providers would come together with the Authority to discuss common issues of interest or concerns. The initial concept was for an Area Forum involving all the providers in an Area, both statutory and voluntary, providing a mechanism for co-operation between providers and allowing each to have an input into the service planning and evaluation processes. It could also be used to bring together providers for a particular care group (the elderly, the disabled, children) or for a particular illness (asthma, heart disease, diabetes). It would cultivate the networks through which primary, acute and community services providers spoke to each other and to the Authority and it could operate at district, area or regional level.

The proposed framework for membership of the Board of the Authority is very much along the lines set out by the Ministerial statement of November 1996, retaining current Eastern Health Board provision for the representation of registered health professionals and for Ministerial nominees, adding new members drawn from voluntary hospitals, the mental handicap agencies and the other voluntary bodies, and increasing the number of public representatives to ensure they hold their majority.

The Area boundaries, as proposed by the Minister, are largely accepted, subject to proposed minor changes. It is suggested that County Kildare be not divided, but that it should in whole form part of the South West Area; that the Area boundary in County Wicklow follow the electoral line of the Baltinglass electoral area; and that the Pembroke Electoral division of Dublin City become part of the South East Area.

For management purposes, it is suggested that each Area be divided up into Districts, each of which will have its own general manager and unit of management. To encourage population identification with their own District, they are proposed to follow as far as possible the new Local Authority Boundaries. Thus, Fingal and South County each become a district; Kildare and West Wicklow (Baltinglass) form a single district; Dun Laoghaire/Rathdown and Pembroke form a single district; and East Wicklow becomes a district. The other districts are formed in Dublin City and are set out along clear, identifiable lines.

The overall proposed structures would provide for the continuation and enhancement of the strengths of the current system and would recognise and respect the traditions, initiatives, experience and skills of hospitals and services, who themselves or whose direct antecedents have been providing services for some hundreds of years. But it would also address the recognised defects and create the framework for co-operation and cohesion, for providing comprehensiveness, integration and holism, and for moving towards the seamless service which patients and clients deserve.

THE OUTCOMES

At the time of writing, the legislation is being drafted and we must await the publication of the Bill and its ultimate enactment in law. But if the final outcome approximates the advice of the Task Force, it is possible to begin to look into the future and assess the likely results.

In some ways, there will not be any great changes in the first year or two. The new Authority will inherit the current services of the Eastern Health Board and the current arrangements which the Department of Health and Children has with the 35 voluntary agencies. Existing budgets will have been fixed for the providers and no dramatic changes are envisaged. Indeed, there is good reason why some steady-state elements should apply, to provide the reassurance and confidence that many will seek in a time of change.

There will, however, be some significant changes, even from A-day. For the first time in the history of the region, there will be a unified comprehensive authority responsible for the co-ordination and funding of all health and social services in the East, both statutory and voluntary. Its work will be informed by information on measured need, its resources will comprise a budget of some £1.3 billion, and its providing agencies will employ some 27,000 staff. It will be required to plan and commission services and to monitor and evaluate their results in the context of the objectives of the Health Strategy: health gain and social gain; health and social status; addressing the big killer diseases and conditions which cause premature death; promoting health; preventing illness; treating the sick; and alleviating personal social problems. In its allocation of resources, it will be charged with responsibility for deciding priority on the basis of the foregoing parameters and of ensuring efficiency, effectiveness and value for money. It will create a forum and head up a framework which will provide the opportunity for the pursuit of excellence in a comprehensive way in the health services. For the first time, there will be an advocate to the Minister on behalf of all the health needs of the Eastern Region and of its providers.

There will also be three Area Councils, each vested with all the powers of a normal Health Board with respect to its own statutory services. Each will be charged with delivering in its own area the full range of services currently delivered by the Eastern Health Board. It will also, as part of its agreement with the Authority, be required to work closely with the voluntary agencies in its Area. It will provide a new forum, closer to the point of delivery of services, in which local priorities and needs can be addressed, decided and delivered. Through its Council members, each of whom is a member of the Authority, and through its Chief Executive, who will work closely with the regional executive, it can feed into the regional planning process. The decentralisation of the work of the Eastern Health Board into these Area Councils means that each Area can now be more responsive to local needs and can provide a mix of services which better meet the priorities of the area. The operational autonomy of these Councils provides the opportunity for innovation and progression at both area and district level.

The voluntary agencies will no longer be a series of a stand-alone service providers, but, while retaining their operational autonomy and their corporate identity, will form part of a framework of care in the East. They will have sectoral representation on the Regional

Authority and on the Area Councils. They will have clear agreements and plans with the central Authority for the services they provide and for the resources they will be allocated. They will work in structured co-operation with other providers in the service. Issues such as bed-blockages, waiting times, waiting lists, accident and emergency and step-down services can be addressed and resolved with an Authority which itself has a statutory responsibility to deal with them.

In each of the other regions of the country, the local Health Board itself provides and funds the vast bulk (in some cases nearly 100 per cent) of the health and social services of the region. It can therefore act as the advocate to Government and Minister on behalf of the region; identify the regional priorities, plan and fund on the basis of measured need, secure and provide new and enhanced services to meet emerging needs, monitor and evaluate outputs and outcomes.

Only the Eastern Region does not have such a body as yet.

The ultimate results of the reorganisation can only be judged by its effect on the services delivered to patients and clients. For example, take an elderly patient who is under general practitioner care; who needs urgent acute geriatric care in an acute hospital (voluntary hospital); who on discharge requires some convalescent care (statutory services); who then needs some continued care (nursing home); who improves and can be discharged home with domiciliary support (statutory) and attendance at a day hospital (voluntary hospital). If this patient can move through this sequence easily and without delays and believes he/she is receiving a unified comprehensive and seamless service — then the system is working for him or her. This will require that each of the providers in this sequence must have their interfaces with their colleague services clearly defined, that each provider understands the other's role and function and that the professionals involved are working together.

With 38 separate providers in the region, it is evident that issues of acceptance/admission of patients and clients to a service and of referral/transfer/discharge to another service are vitally important. This issue will become one of the litmus tests of success for the new arrangements.

The setting up of these new structures will provide the opportunity for new and innovative thinking to be introduced into the Irish Health Services. This work is being paralleled in Scandinavia and in Britain and interest is being taken in the work of the Task Force in many European cities, who are themselves exploring new models to create a better environment and framework for the work of hospitals and the wider health and social services. We in turn can learn from their work in building on the new structures that this reorganisation will create.

The implementation of these new arrangements will, I believe, open up a new exciting and challenging chapter in the long history of the health services in the region, and will go a long way to solve what the Health Strategy called "a particular problem in the East . . ."

4

HEALTH EXPENDITURE TRENDS IN IRELAND: PAST, PRESENT AND FUTURE

Miriam M. Wiley

INTRODUCTION

There is no "right" answer to the question of what level of resources should be invested in a health care system. Over the past two decades, many countries have invested considerable effort in attempting to shed light on this question (Stationery Office, 1989; OECD, 1992). One result of these investigations is an increasing recognition that any attempt to quantify the "right" level of resources for health service investment may provide the least productive starting point for an informed discussion on this question. It may be more appropriate to initiate such a discussion through consideration of the level of resources that may be considered "affordable" for the support of any country's health care system. In this chapter, the resource commitment which has been considered "affordable" for the Irish health care system in recent decades will be reviewed. In addition to looking at past patterns of expenditure, the factors which may be expected to influence expenditure levels into the next millennium will also be assessed.

The Irish health service is predominantly a tax-funded system. The overall funding level for the health services is determined in negotiations between the Department of Finance and the Department of Health and Children, which provides annual budgets to the eight regional health boards for the provision of public health services. Funding is also provided to the voluntary hospitals and other service delivery agencies in the voluntary sector. Health service budgets are determined by demographic factors, commitments to service provision, national pay policies and the general economic guidelines applied to the operation of the public service as a whole. In addition to service delivery agencies, other corporate bodies and registration boards such as the Blood Transfusion Service Board are supported by the Department of Health and Children.

While the Irish health system continues to be funded primarily from the central exchequer, the proportion of total expenditure derived from public sources has been declining. In the 1980s, the central exchequer contributed approximately 85 per cent of total health expenditure, compared with a current contribution level of around 75 per cent. Approximately one-quarter of total health expenditure now consists of expenditure from private sources, particularly from health insurance companies and household expenditure on general practitioner visits, pharmaceuticals and private hospital stays. The tax-funded share of public health expenditure has also dropped over this period from a level of 87.9 per cent in 1980 to 82.4 per cent in 1996. While part of this decline has been offset by the introduction of user charges for public health services in 1987, the share of health expenditure funded from other sources, including the National Lottery, EU receipts and local income, increased by 3.2 per cent over this period (OECD, 1997).

In reviewing variations in Irish health expenditure over time, clear patterns can be observed in the changes occurring in particular periods. In the next section, variations in health expenditure in the period preceding the 1990s will be reviewed, followed by an exploration of developments in the current decade to date. The lessons of past experience for the anticipation of health expenditure trends into the next millennium will then be considered.

IRISH HEALTH EXPENDITURE: PRE-1990S

In each of the four decades following the establishment of the Department of Health in 1947, the share of GNP devoted to health expenditure increased by over 30 per cent (Wiley, 1997). While the first decade of the Department of Health's existence was associated with the greatest increase in health expenditure relative to GNP, the most recent period of expansion can be traced to the 1970s. In this decade, the proportion of GNP allocated to health increased by 56.8 per cent, from 4.4 per cent in 1970/71 to 6.9 per cent in 1979. During this period, public spending increased substantially and health service eligibility and availability were also expanded.

Developments in the 1980s were, however, in sharp contrast to the 1970s, as a public expenditure crisis and economic recession were associated with a reduction of 16 per cent in the proportion of GNP allocated to health expenditure from 8.1 per cent in 1980 to 6.8 per cent in 1989. The decline in health expenditure over this period is evident in Figure 4.1, which shows gross non-capital health expenditure in current and constant terms (1990 prices) and as a percentage of GDP and GNP since 1980. In addition to a reduction in the proportion of GNP and GDP allocated to health, between 1980 and 1989, gross non-capital health expenditure in constant terms (1990 prices) actually dropped by 4.2 per cent. The pressure on health expenditure throughout the 1980s was quite exceptional following the expansionism of the 1970s and preceding the very different economic experience in the Ireland of the 1990s.

Figure 4.1: Gross Non-Capital Health Expenditure in Current and Constant Terms and as a Percentage of GNP and GDP: 1980-1997

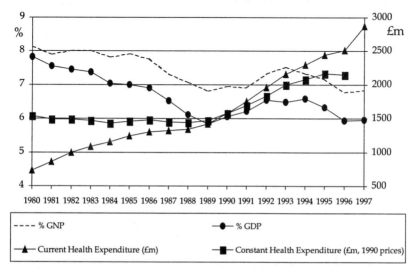

Source: Department of Health and Children estimates, 1998.

IRISH HEALTH EXPENDITURE IN THE 1990S

If one were to focus simply on the share of GNP or GDP devoted to health, trends in the 1990s would, at a superficial level, not look very different from previous years. The decade began with close to seven per cent of GNP being devoted to gross non-capital health expenditure, an estimate which increased to a high of 7.5 per cent in 1993. There has been a general downward trend since then, to the point where 6.6 per cent of GNP was allocated to gross non-capital health expenditure in 1998.[1] The net result of these changes is that, since the beginning of the 1990s, there has been a 5.3 per cent reduction in the proportion of GNP devoted to gross non-capital health expenditure.

It is, however, necessary to look behind these trends to get the true picture of developments in the Irish economy this decade. To enable some understanding of these developments, changes in GNP and GDP, together with gross non-capital health expenditure in current and constant terms, are presented in Figure 4.2.

Figure 4.2: Gross National Product, Gross Domestic Product and Gross Non-Capital Health Expenditure in Current and Constant Terms: 1980–1997

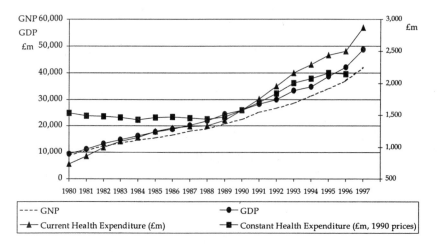

---

[1] Estimate provided by the Department of Health and Children.

In summary, the 1990s has been a decade of exceptional growth in the Irish economy with average annual GNP growth (at constant market prices) between 1991 and 1997 estimated at 6.3 per cent (CSO, 1998). This contrasts with average annual GNP growth (at constant market prices) of 3.6 per cent between 1984 and 1990 (CSO, 1991). While the share of GNP/GDP devoted to gross non-capital health expenditure has shown a decline over the 1990s as a whole, because of the growth in the economy, this expenditure has actually been increasing in real terms. Between 1990 and 1996, gross non-capital health expenditure in constant terms (at 1990 prices) increased by 36 per cent. It is interesting that since 1993, when the share of GNP devoted to health began to decline, gross non-capital health expenditure in constant terms actually increased by seven per cent.

To facilitate an understanding of the experience of different sectors with changes in health expenditure levels, Figure 4.3 shows the distribution of public health expenditure by programme between 1980 and 1994. The proportion of public health expenditure allocated to the general and special hospitals programmes generally decreased over this period. The share of total expenditure allocated to the general hospital programme dropped from a level of 53.8 per cent in 1980 to 50.1 per cent in 1994, while the special hospital programme accounted for 20.9 per cent of public health expenditure in 1980, compared with 19.1 per cent in 1994. This contrasts with the growth in the community care programme from a level of 20.5 per cent in 1980 to 26.8 per cent in 1994. It is interesting that it is this health expenditure programme covering community health, welfare, protection and services for the handicapped which accounted for the largest proportional increase between 1990 and 1994. Over this period, the community care programme grew by over 12 per cent annually, compared with an annual increase of 9 per cent in the public hospital programme (OECD, 1997). This reflects a consistent trend since the early 1980s of a reduction in the share of health expenditure allocated to hospital services and an increase in investment in the community care area.

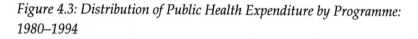

Figure 4.3: Distribution of Public Health Expenditure by Programme: 1980–1994

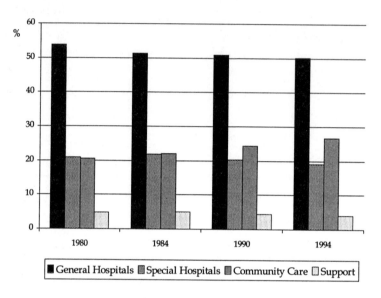

In summary, the Irish experience can be considered quite unusual in international terms, as a declining share of GNP devoted to health in the 1980s was associated with a real cut in gross non-capital health expenditure, while real increases in health expenditure in the 1990s also command a smaller share of GNP due to the high rate of growth in the economy in general. The Irish experience in the international context will be considered in more detail in the next section.

THE INTERNATIONAL PERSPECTIVE

The evolution of health expenditure in recent decades in Ireland is increasingly appearing quite unique in a European context. Table 4.1 shows total health expenditure as a proportion of Gross Domestic Product (GDP) for EU member states for selected years between 1980 and 1996, together with changes in this indicator over the period (OECD Health Data, 1998). At 8.7 per cent in 1980, Ireland ranked joint third relative to other EU member states in terms of the share of GDP devoted to health. The Irish and Danish level at the time was exceeded by Sweden, with over 9 per cent of GDP allocated to health expenditure, and Germany, with 8.8 per cent. While Sweden and Germany ranked as the biggest spenders on health throughout the 1980s, the Irish estimates show that the rank occupied by Ireland was progressively declining, as the proportion of GDP devoted to health in Ireland ranked joint fifth relative to other member states in 1985 and eleventh in 1990. Since 1993, the only EU member states to spend a smaller proportion of GDP on health are the United Kingdom, Luxembourg and Greece.

Table 4.1: Total Expenditure on Health as a Percentage of GDP for EU Member States, 1980–96

	%				Percentage Change (%)			
	1980	1985	1990	1996	1980–85	1985–90	1990–96	1980–96
Austria	7.7	6.7	7.2	8.0	–12.99	7.46	11.11	3.90
Belgium	6.5	7.3	7.5	7.8	12.31	2.74	4.00	20.00
Denmark	8.7	8.2	8.2	8.0	–5.75	0.00	–2.44	–8.05
Finland	6.5	7.3	8.0	7.4	12.31	9.59	–7.50	13.85
France	7.6	8.5	8.9	9.7	11.84	4.71	8.99	27.63
Germany	8.8	9.3	8.7	10.5	5.68	-6.45	20.69	19.32
Greece	3.6	4.0	4.2	6.8	11.11	5.00	61.90	88.89
Ireland	8.7	7.9	6.7	7.0	–9.20	–15.19	4.48	–19.54
Italy	7.0	7.1	8.1	7.8	1.43	14.08	–3.70	11.43
Luxembourg	6.2	6.1	6.6	6.8	–1.61	8.20	3.03	9.68
Netherlands	7.9	7.9	8.3	8.6	0.00	5.06	3.61	8.86
Portugal	5.8	6.3	6.5	8.3	8.62	3.17	27.69	43.10
Spain	5.6	5.6	6.9	7.4	0.00	23.21	7.25	32.14
Sweden	9.4	9.0	8.8	8.6	–4.26	–2.22	–2.27	–8.51
United Kingdom	5.6	5.9	6.0	6.9	5.36	1.69	15.00	23.21

Source: OECD Health Data, 1998.

Table 4.1 also shows the percentage change in the share of GDP allocated to health for the periods 1980–85, 1985–90, 1990–96 and 1980–96. Between 1980 and 1985, five countries show a reduction in the proportion of GDP allocated to health expenditure, with the biggest reduction shown for Austria at 13 per cent followed by Ireland at 9 per cent. This contrasts with increases of over 11 per cent for Belgium, Finland, France and Greece over the same period. Between 1985 and 1990, only three countries show a reduction in this indicator. The biggest reduction of 15 per cent in the proportion of GDP devoted to health is estimated for Ireland, with reductions of 7 per cent and 2 per cent, respectively, for Germany and Sweden. For the same period, the largest increase is shown for Spain at over 23 per cent, followed by 14 per cent for Italy. The period 1990–96 showed substantial and contrasting changes, with four countries reporting reductions of between 2 and 8 per cent in the levels of GDP allocated to health while the estimates for Greece, Portugal, Germany[2] and the UK increased by 62 per cent, 28 per cent, 21 per cent and 15 per cent respectively. When the whole 1980–96 period is assessed, only three EU member states show a reduction in the allocation to health, with by far the biggest reduction of 20 per cent shown for Ireland, followed by Sweden at 9 per cent and Denmark at 8 per cent. Of the 12 countries showing a rise in health expenditure relative to GDP, the biggest increase is estimated for Greece at 89 per cent, followed by Portugal at 43 per cent, Spain at 32 per cent, France at 27 per cent, the UK at 23 per cent and Belgium and Germany at around 20 per cent.

To provide a picture of current levels of expenditure in EU member states, Figure 4.4 presents the proportion of GDP devoted to health for 1995 and 1996. For both years, Germany and France are consistently the biggest spenders with close to ten per cent of GDP committed to health expenditure. Only four countries spend seven per cent or less of GDP on health, i.e. Greece, Ireland, Luxembourg and the UK. The share of GDP devoted to health between 1995 and 1996 increased in six countries, dropped in five countries and re-

---

[2] The unification of Germany must be acknowledged as an important factor contributing to the increased levels of health expenditure.

mained stable in four countries over the period. Given the previous and current experience nationally and internationally, the next section will consider the factors which might be expected to influence future trends in commitments to expenditure on the health services in Ireland.

Figure 4.4: Total Health Expenditure as a Percentage of GDP for EU Member States: 1995 and 1996

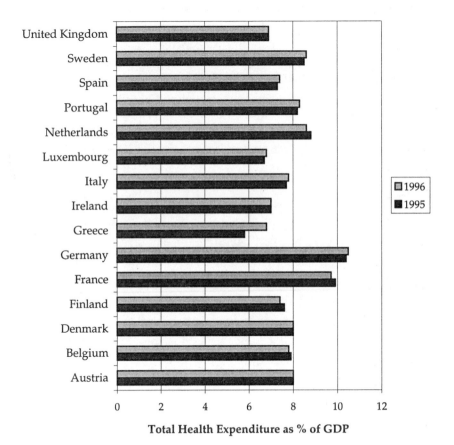

Total Health Expenditure as % of GDP

Source: OECD Health Data, 1998.

FUTURE DEVELOPMENTS FOR IRISH HEALTH EXPENDITURE

As the blueprint for the development of the modern Irish health services, the White Paper in 1966 demonstrated impressive foresight and a number of observations continue to be as relevant today as they were three decades ago. The following statement with regard to the financing of the health services in the latter decades of the twentieth century continues to be relevant to planned development into the next millennium:

> The government fully accept that those employed in the health services should benefit from periodic rounds of pay increases, in the same way as others in public employment, and recognise that rises in the cost of the services will follow this. There are other factors, too, which continually tend to augment the cost of the services, including the increasing complexity of medicine, better standards of staffing, rises in prices of drugs and medical requisites . . . and the increasing cost of maintaining the fabric of institutions and the equipment in them. Therefore if there were to be no further developments or expansion in the health services, health expenditure would continue to inexorably rise (Department of Health, 1966: 58).

What is particularly important about the view expressed here is a recognition of the difficulty of holding health expenditure constant when the inherent tendency of many of the key influences on health expenditure levels is to exert pressure for expansion. This pressure for expansion is exerted by such factors as public sector pay levels and employment, advances in medical technology, changes in health service consumption patterns, demographic developments, etc. The real cuts in health expenditure which occurred in the 1980s were achieved in the context of a public service employment embargo and pay pause, a declining birth rate, high emigration and the most widespread programme of hospital closures ever undertaken in this country. These would have to be considered extreme measures in an economy in recession and are indicative of the efforts which are required to achieve real cuts in health expenditure.

While the economic boom in the Ireland of the late 1990s may not continue into perpetuity, it is reasonable to assume that the experience of the 1980s was exceptional and the draconian measures required to achieve real cuts in health expenditure are unlikely to be revisited on the Irish health services. Given the inherent pressure for expansion, therefore, the question that remains to be addressed is which level of increase in health expenditure may be considered affordable in the short to medium term. Any response to this question will necessitate consideration of the range of influences contributing to this expansionary pressure. Many of these factors are explored in detail by other contributors to this publication and a brief review of the issues arising will be presented here (Barry, 1998; Dwyer and Taaffe, 1998; Fahey, 1998; Gul and Darzi, 1998; Swanwick and Lawlor, 1998).

As public sector pay constitutes the largest component of health expenditure, the scope of any future national agreements between the social partners will have direct implications for resource requirements in health, together with other areas of the public sector. While public sector pay levels may be outside the specific control of the health sector, the numbers employed are determined by this sector and directly contribute to the size of the overall pay bill. Current trends indicate an increase in total employment in the health services. Between 1990 and 1996, there was an increase of 9.9 per cent in total health personnel employment compared with an increase of 5.1 per cent over the 1980–89 period. In total, there was an increase of 18.3 per cent in the numbers employed in the health services between 1980 and 1996 (OECD Health Data, 1998). As a contributor to overall health expenditure, therefore, the public sector pay component can be expected to continue to increase in the foreseeable future.

Technological and pharmaceutical advances will always challenge the boundaries of medical science. While these developments may not be expected to contribute to substantial increases in life expectancy in the short term, areas most likely to be affected include service and treatment options for particular conditions, quality of life experience and the level of avoidable and treatable morbidity. Advances in treatment options may also directly contribute to increases in the volume of services consumed. A very interesting example of this phenomenon is provided by the growth of day care within the acute hospital sector in Ireland. While the number of acute hospital beds remained stable between 1990 and 1997, the number of inpatients treated increased by 4.1 per cent and the number of day cases doubled to a level of one-quarter of a million (Department of

Health and Children estimates, 1998). In this case, the improvements in technology enabled a shift in site of care from inpatient to day care for many treatment and investigative procedures. This resulted in a 23 per cent increase in the number of people treated within the acute care sector between 1990 and 1997, even though the number of hospital beds available remained the same. When technological innovation and increased utilisation of services are combined with rising consumer expectations and concerns about medico-legal issues, it is reasonable to expect further increases in both the range and volume of health services consumed within the Irish system (Cusack, 1998).

What emerges clearly from this review of expenditure trends in recent decades is that public investment in the Irish health services is generally reflective of the wellbeing of the Irish economy as a whole. This is not particularly unusual and supports the view that expenditure on health is closely related to the level of investment which can be supported economically and politically. Any attempt to assess future trends must therefore have regard to medium-term projections for the economy as a whole. The ESRI's medium-term forecast for 1997–2003 suggests that the current exceptional rate of growth in the Irish economy is likely to continue into the next decade, assuming the continuation of prudent fiscal policy, wage moderation and the absence of serious domestic or international shocks (Duffy et al., 1997). Given a continuation of current growth rates, the *Review* predicts that "Ireland will approach the EU average standard of living around the middle of the next decade, probably exceeding that of the UK before 2005" (p. vii). In such circumstances, it is likely that health expenditure levels will continue to rise into the new millennium. As public health expenditure as a proportion of GNP has been held below eight per cent since 1984, this trend would be expected to continue given the growth in GNP forecast for the next decade (Duffy et al., 1997).

CONCLUSION

In analysing the current strengths and weaknesses of the Irish health system, the Department of Health's strategy document, *Shaping a Healthier Future*, recognises the importance of the prevailing political and social consensus for the development of an adequately funded, high-quality and equitable public system (Department of Health, 1994). Additional attributes noted include the well-qualified, committed and caring staff, the strong voluntary sector and the mix of public and private services fulfilling complementary roles. This view is supported by a recent review undertaken by the OECD which concluded that "The Irish health system is based on a mixture of public and private care which has resulted in good provision of health care at relatively low cost to the taxpayer" (OECD, 1997: 150).

It is, however, also recognised that weaknesses persist within the health system and *Shaping a Healthier Future* suggests that these include the fact that the main causes of premature mortality have not been adequately addressed; many services are not targeted towards the achievement of specific goals; and co-ordination, organisation and management within the system generally are less than adequate (Department of Health, 1994). In addition, the OECD propose that "The principal problems facing the health services in Ireland appear to be related to the control of spending and ensuring that resources are used and allocated efficiently" (OECD, 1997: 142). All of the indications emerging from this review of health expenditure trends, however, suggest that expenditure levels will continue to increase through to the next decade in the absence of explicit spending controls. Even if wage moderation is supported within the public sector in the medium term, growth in the size of health sector employment, together with increases in the range and volume of services consumed, would be expected to exert continuing pressure for growth in health expenditure levels into the next millennium.

The annual resource investment in the Irish health services, like other health systems internationally, can be considered a political decision. It therefore seems reasonable to assume that societal priorities for the investment of productive resources are reflected in this decision. If the prioritisation of health system requirements in the Irish context is considered worthy of the anticipated growth in health expenditure levels, in conclusion it may be worth noting the cautionary advice offered by the architects of the modern health services when considering the implications of further development:

... our health services ... must be planned so as to ensure the utmost efficiency and economy in their administration and so as to avoid expenditure on services (or extensions of services) not demonstrated to be reasonably necessary (Department of Health, 1966: 26).

References

Barry, J. (1998), "Developments in the Epidemiology of Disease in the Next Century", this volume.

Central Statistics Office (1991), *National Income and Expenditure 1990*, Dublin: Stationery Office, November.

CSO (1998), *National Income and Expenditure 1997*, Dublin: Stationery Office, July.

Cusack, D. (1998), "Risk Management as a Strategy for Quality", this volume.

Department of Health (1966), *The Health Service and their Future Development*, White Paper, Dublin: Stationery Office.

Department of Health (1994), *Shaping a Healthier Future: A Strategy for Effective Healthcare in the 1990s*, Dublin: Stationery Office.

Duffy, D., J. Fitzgerald, I. Kearney and F. Shortall (1997), *Medium-Term Review: 1997–2003*, Dublin: The Economic and Social Research Institute, April.

Dwyer, M. and P. Taaffe (1998), "Nursing in 21st Century Ireland: Opportunities for Transformation", this volume.

Fahey, T. (1998), "Population Ageing, the Elderly and Health Care", this volume.

Gul, Y. and A. Darzi (1998), "Development and Assessment of Medical Technology", this volume.

OECD (1992), *The Reform of Health Care: A Comparative Analysis of Seven OECD Countries*, Health Policy Studies, No. 2, Paris: OECD.

OECD Health Data (1998), Paris: OECD.

OECD (1997), *Economic Surveys 1996–1997: Ireland*, Paris: OECD.

Stationery Office (1989), *Report of the Commission on Health Funding*, Dublin: Stationery Office.

Swanwick, G. and B. Lawlor (1998), "Services for Dementia Sufferers and Their Carers: Implications for Future Development", this volume.

Wiley, Miriam M. (1997), "Irish Health Policy in Perspective" in F. O' Muircheartaigh (ed.), *Ireland in the Coming Times*, Dublin: Institute of Public Administration.

5

THE FUTURE POLITICAL, LEGISLATIVE AND SOCIAL FRAMEWORK OF THE HEALTH SERVICES

Ruth Barrington

INTRODUCTION

The political and legislative framework for the health services for the 21st century is likely to develop gradually in response to the challenges facing the health services over the next few decades. That has been the pattern of the past — change and continuity in creative tension. It is difficult to predict the exact challenges or to give relative weightings to issues that will influence this framework. This chapter suggests some issues facing the health services, the resolution of which will change the political and legislative framework of tomorrow's health services.

The health services are intricately interwoven with the fabric of Irish life. They are subjected to the same forces that operate on Irish life in general and on the public service in particular. They deal in a commodity — health — to which people have always attached importance but which, with the improvement in the health of the population over the past 50 years, has grown in their priorities. Health and the issues that surround it arouse strong passions, for a number of reasons. The extent to which good health is enjoyed by everyone in a society, regardless of economic or social circumstances or gender is an important indicator of how much that society values equality. Because the health services deal with issues of life and death, fertility and reproduction and the interface between technology and human nature, its problems are never simple. The health services touch every home in the country, with millions of interactions taking place each year. The health services are major employers, employing over 66,000 people in 1996, and many others depend for a living on the business of health and illness (Department of Health and Children, 1996). In 1998, the taxpayer will contribute £2.6 billion to the cost of running the health services, amounting to 25 per cent of public expenditure (Department of Finance, 1998).

It is useful to consider the influences shaping the political and legislative structure of the health services under a number of headings. The health services have objectives that are unique to health but they also have a responsibility to assist in the achievement of others. The core objective of the health services is greater health and social gain for the population by prevention of disease, promotion of health, the treatment of disease, support for the disabled and the protection of the welfare of children.

In addition to what might be called the core role of the health service, it has a contribution to make to wider objectives of the society in which it operates. These objectives include contributing to the economic and social development of the country, to making Ireland a more democratic, open and transparent society, to better government in this country and to the creation of peace on this island. The development of what might be called the core and secondary roles of the health services will in turn influence the political and legislative framework in which the health services will operate in the next century. Before examining likely developments under each of these headings, a brief analysis is made of the current framework.

CURRENT POLITICAL AND LEGISLATIVE FRAMEWORK

The health services operate in the framework of a parliamentary democracy, the rules of which are set out in the Constitution and laws passed by the Oireachtas. The Constitution and the laws made under it set out the rights of citizens, the responsibilities of public bodies towards the citizens they serve and the limits of the powers they can exercise. Within Government, the Minister for Health and Children is assigned responsibility for the management of the Department of Health and Children and is answerable to the Oireachtas for his or her stewardship. The Department of Health and Children is responsible for the development of policy on health, the translation of that policy where necessary into law, securing finances from the Exchequer to fund the health services and the efficient use of resources in the health services. In recent years, the priorities for health of each incoming government have been set out in programmes for government.[1] Priorities are also set by the process of social partnership that result in the national agreements on economic and social progress.[2]

The entitlements of people to health services and responsibilities to protect health are set out in the Health Acts, 1947–1996. The responsibility to provide health services lies principally with the eight health boards and also with specialised agencies that provide services that are better organised at a national level, such as the Irish Medicines Board or the Blood Transfusion Board.

The health services, as they developed in this country, were principally the responsibility of local authorities in which locally elected representatives decided on the amount of local taxation to be raised to pay for the services provided. After the Second World War, there was an intense desire to improve the health of the people and the link between local representation and local taxation was seen as a constraint on the development of better health services (detailed in Barrington, 1987). In 1947, national Government agreed to pay a contribution towards the cost of health services locally until it reached the same amount as the amount being spent in each county. However, by the late 1960s, the cost of the expanded health services had grown so rapidly that the removal of health charges from local taxation had become a major political issue.[3] At the same time, the Government had decided to establish a regional structure to replace the county system, principally to facilitate the emergence of a regional hospital system. The Health Act, 1970, established eight health

---

[1] The programme of the Fianna Fáil/Progressive Democrat Government, which took office in June 1997, is "An Action Programme for the Millennium".

[2] The current programme agreed between the Government and the social partners is Partnership 2000.

[3] The financing of the health services is examined in detail by Wiley (1997).

boards, transferring the responsibilities previously exercised by the counties and a number of larger health authorities. In 1974, the Government decided to remove health charges from local taxation and to fund expenditure on the health services entirely from the Exchequer. (Chapter 1 discusses the structure of the health boards and the health system in general.)

The membership of the health boards, which maintained the principle of democratic accountability by having a majority of public representatives, was expanded to include elected members of the registered professions working in the health services and appointees of the Minister for Health. The removal of responsibility for raising even a small share of the funding for the health services in each region from local taxation or even regional taxation, coupled with strong pressure to improve the health services from the electorate and the professions, created a dynamic in favour of rapid increases in expenditure on services in the 1970s and early 1980s. The rapid increase in expenditure was halted in the late 1980s but only when the overall Exchequer situation became critical.

In the early 1990s, the Government expressed its concern not to return to what was seen as the bad old days of overspending by the health boards. The issue was how to make health boards more financially accountable. The response was the Health (Amendment) (No.2) Act, 1996, that requires the health boards to operate within tight policy and financial procedures. A sharp distinction has been drawn in the Act, similar to that in local government legislation, between the executive functions of the chief executive officer of the board and the policy-making role of the members. However, the Act does not restore the link between local or regional taxation and representation that at the end of the day is the most effective way of encouraging responsible decision-making in a democracy.

Despite the financial challenge, the health boards remain the most developed regional bodies in terms of the majority of public representatives in the membership, the scale of their functions and budgets and the number of employees. The involvement of public representatives is critical to their success. Decision-making in the health services is about balancing interests with the goal of improving the quality of life of some or all of the people. Decisions on health services touch on the most sensitive issues of people's lives. They may affect their businesses or the value of their properties, the prestige of their towns or the safety of their neighbourhoods. A proposal to change the use of a hospital, to locate a hostel for the mentally ill in a residential neighbourhood, to provide a sterilisation service or to develop a special care unit for disturbed children can arouse the deepest of emotions and, in a democracy with a free media, must be handled with skill and diplomacy. The involvement of politicians, whose job is to balance interests in the public good, is critical to getting a consensus on issues or at least to diffusing conflict. If a mechanism is not built in which allows these issues to be resolved through local or regional structures, they will surface at national level, making it even more difficult for a Minister to concentrate on performing essential tasks. Calls to "take politics out of health" — usually made by members of the medical profession who cannot understand why the technocratic answer is not the one the politicians immediately favour — are wide of the mark because they misunderstand the nature of decision-making in the health services.

The relationship between the Minister and the Department has also been affected in recent times by legislation. The Public Service Management Act, 1997, does not alter the fundamental responsibility of the Minister for the activities or non-action of the Department, but it does encourage more explicit recognition of the Department in the management of the responsibilities for which it is responsible. The Act sets out for the first time the responsibilities of the secretary-general of a department. Each department is required by the Public Service Management Act to present to the Minister a statement of strategy within six months of the Minister taking up duty and, if he or she remains in office, three years from the date of the previous statement. This statement, it should be emphasised, is primarily about the priorities of the Department within the health system. It complements but does not supersede *Shaping a Healthier Future — a Strategy for Effective Health Care in the 1990s*, which, as its name implies, is addressed to the health services in general (Department of Health, 1994). The Minister has announced that *Shaping a Healthier*

Future will be reviewed and updated to provide a strategic direction for the health services as a whole in the first decade of the new century.[4]

The Freedom of Information Act, 1997, is also having a profound effect on the management and organisation of the Department. A culture that protected information on the basis that to disclose it might be inimical to the interests of the Minister must now cope with a culture in which a citizen has a right to information, a right that can only be refused on certain limited grounds. It is too early yet to be definitive on the impact of the Act on government departments but it is likely to have a significant impact on those departments whose services touch on issues of vital concern to citizens. Health is one of those departments.

The voluntary bodies that provide services on behalf of the Department or the health boards are another important part of the structure of health services. From the large teaching hospitals owned by religious orders to small parents' associations running services for people with a mental handicap, voluntary organisations bring a depth and richness to the organisation and provision of health services. The majority of voluntary organisations receive funding for the services they provide from the health boards, but the voluntary hospitals and some mental handicap agencies have received their funding direct from the Department. *Shaping a Healthier Future* announced a change in this relationship with the Department, while guaranteeing the operational autonomy and independent identity of the voluntary agencies. Work is currently under way to replace the funding relationship with the Department with a more satisfactory relationship with the health boards. In the greater Dublin area, a new health authority will replace the Eastern Health Board and take over responsibility for funding those agencies funded direct by the Department. The report, *Enhancing the Partnership*, set out the framework in which funding of the mental handicap agencies is transferring to health boards (Department of Health and Children, 1997b). The con-

---

[4] Mr Brian Cowen TD, Minister for Health, address at the launch of *Reflections on Health*, op. cit, Royal College of Physicians on 19 November 1997.

tractual relationships of the larger voluntary organisations with the health boards will be formalised in service agreements, which will replace the current, rather *ad hoc*, arrangements.

The specialist health agencies are another sector of the health services that are experiencing great change, if not trauma, at the present time. Specialist health agencies are those bodies that have been established to provide a specialised service on a national basis, such as the Food Safety Authority and the Blood Transfusion Board, or to carry out a task that is better done on a national basis, such as the regulation of the professions. The disastrous contamination of the anti-D product with the hepatitis C virus by the Blood Transfusion Board and the consequent infection of 1,500 persons, mainly women, with the virus, has highlighted the responsibilities on every health agency to ensure the highest standards of safety in its operations. Protection of the public is increasingly demanded as a primary objective of the bodies that regulate the professions, such as the Medical Council and An Bord Altranais, a demand that is increasingly likely to be reflected explicitly in legislation.

ACHIEVING HEALTH AND SOCIAL GAIN

The primary goal of the health services is to increase health and social gain in the community. The health services have traditionally achieved their goals by prevention (vaccination, inspection of food), by the provision of curative and therapeutic services and by support for children and adults with disabilities and in dysfunctional families. By far the most developed of the above are the curative services, which employ most people, are the most expensive to provide and are at the leading edge of technology. As well as being essential when acute medical care is required, they have also transformed the lives of people who would otherwise have been condemned to a poor quality of life. Joint replacement, cataract surgery and coronary artery by-pass, just to mention the best known treatments, have transformed the lives of thousands of people for the better.

The success of curative medicine can sometimes lead to an assumption, however, that more medical care is the most effective way of increasing health and social gain at the end of the 20th century. It may not be. The major killers in this country now, as in most of western Europe, are cardiovascular disease, cancer and accidents. All three are associated with multiple causes. Their causes lie deep within the way in which we collectively and individually order our lives. They are influenced by the food we eat, whether or not we smoke, take enough exercise, live with abnormal levels of stress, how fast we drive and how we order our system of transport.

These diseases and accidents pose a challenge to our society, not just to the health services. The health sector, because it understands the nature and causes of these diseases, and because health professionals are too aware that curative services can have little more than a palliative effect on these diseases, must find a framework in which to reorder individual and collective behaviour for health. The major gains in health in the next century in this country will come from reducing premature deaths from heart disease and cancer and lessening deaths and injuries on our roads. The gains in mental health will come from ensuring that people have the skills to cope with the problems of life and that they feel they are valued members of their communities. Encouraging people to lead healthier and safer lives and providing them with an environment in which to do so requires a partnership for health that goes far beyond present structures or legislation. The extent to which an effective framework can be put in place to achieve these objectives will perhaps be the most important step in achieving greater health for our people in the next century.

The challenge posed by the inter-sectoral nature of our health problems was recognised in the 1980s (Health Education Bureau, 1987). A Cabinet subcommittee was to be established to pull together, at the highest level, the departments with the greatest impact on health, but it was short-lived. The Department's Health Promotion Strategy led to the establishment of the Health Promotion Council, on which a wide range of statutory and voluntary interests are represented to create a coalition for health (Department of Health, 1995).

One of the first and best examples of inter-sectoral co-operation for health has been in education. Influencing young peoples' attitudes for health was identified early on as a priority and much work has been done by the Department of Health and Children and the Department of Education and Science in preparing curricula on health and related issues.

An inter-sectoral approach is being pushed from other directions too. The concern about the safety of food and the quality of our food exports has brought the issue to the forefront of public debate. The new Food Safety Authority is an example of an inter-sectoral approach to reassure consumers at home and abroad about food safety.

The WHO has argued that the environment in which people live is a major determinant of health. Under a WHO initiative, each member state is in the process of preparing a national environment and health action plan (NEHAP), to ensure that the two sectors work towards the same objectives of a safe and healthy living and working environment.[5] The Irish NEHAP is in preparation and will be published towards the end of 1998 or in early 1999.

An inter-sectoral approach is vital not only at national but also at regional and local levels. The fragmented nature of our governmental system makes such co-operation difficult, especially at regional and local level. The competencies of local authorities and health boards are limited. Many services that touch on health are organised nationally and boundaries, with the exception of those used by local authorities and health boards, vary to an extraordinary extent. Even if a local community wished to organise itself for health, it would find itself facing an organisational bird's nest, the penetration of which would put off even the bravest heart. It would be so much easier if government activity in a particular county or region were channelled through multi-competent regional or local authority bodies that were clearly responsible for development of their areas and the wellbeing, including the health, of their citizens.

A deepening and widening of the inter-sectoral approach to increasing health, both at national level and at the regional and local level, will grow in importance in the next century. An increasingly

---

[5] WHO, Declaration of Helsinki (1994). The aim is that all WHO member states in the European region will have adopted an NEHAP before the Conference on Environment and Health in London in 1999.

sophisticated electorate will demand no less. It is only a matter of time before every premature death on the roads or preventable death from cancer or cardiovascular disease will command the same kind of public attention as deaths from meningitis do today. The health sector needs to anticipate this development and position itself as best it can to influence public policy for health.

CONTRIBUTING TO ECONOMIC AND SOCIAL DEVELOPMENT

The role of education in laying the foundations of the 1990s economic boom is often mentioned, but the contribution of the health services is seldom acknowledged. The success of the health services in controlling the many diseases that destroyed or undermined the health of children meant that they were able to take full advantage of the gradual widening of educational opportunities that opened for them from the 1960s onwards. A good health service is also critical to maintaining a healthy workforce and to making this country an attractive place in which to spend one's life and raise children. It has also been a factor in attracting back to Ireland workers who emigrated when young. The control of endemic diseases and the availability of medical services that are as good as any in the world has also been a factor in attracting foreign investment to Ireland and in marketing this country as a major tourist centre. The health services are not just an added extra when it comes to the economic and social development of this country. They are an integral part of Ireland's economic and social success in recent years.

Despite concerns about the increase in the cost of the health services and the share of GDP consumed by health services, the most recent analysis suggests that the Irish health service is one of the most cost-effective in any OECD country (OECD, 1997). Judicious investment in health services, too often seen as a burden on the economy, would be more appropriately seen as an investment in the economic and social infrastructure of the country. An added bonus is that, since health services are organised and delivered close to where people live, investment in the health services tends to be an investment in every county in the country. The Western Health Board, for example, is the largest employer in the west of Ireland, and the health services provide employment for some of the best-educated and trained people.

The biggest challenge for the health services in the field of economic and social development is the contribution it can make to the reduction of inequality in our society. Poor health is both a result of inequality and a contributory factor to the perpetuation of inequality. People who are poor have worse health than those who are better off and people who have bad health tend to be poorer than those with better health (WHO, 1997). There is a vicious cycle in relation to poverty and health that cries out to be addressed. The WHO goal of "health for all" is a radical challenge to member states to take action (WHO, 1984; WHO, forthcoming). The extent of inequality of health in this country between the least and most disadvantaged groups appears to be greater than in other comparable countries.[6]

The response of the health services to the health problems associated with poverty and disadvantage has tended to be palliative. The patient's symptoms are treated but little is done to address the underlying problems giving rise to health problems in the first place. It is not the job of the health services, some would argue, to address problems of inadequate income, overcrowding, violence in the home or neighbourhood and unemployment. However, one must always be aware that policies intended to achieve one purpose may have the unintended effect of contributing to the perpetuation of disadvantage. There is concern, for example, that the income guidelines for a medical card, which roughly coincide with the income of families that are unemployed, act as a disincentive to people to enter or re-enter the workforce. The medical card is especially important to families on low incomes, because it is a passport to other free services, apart from medical care.

The good news is that the health services are increasingly involved in addressing some of the problems that contribute to poor health among those on low incomes. The more proactive approach

---

[6] *The Journal of Health Gain*, Vol. 1, No. 1, June 1997, summarises the information available on health inequalities.

by health boards to promoting family planning, for example, is of vital importance to women on low incomes who wish to control their fertility. The development of counselling, part funded by health boards, has also helped many women to assert themselves and to deal with personal and family problems. The community mothers scheme initiated by the Eastern Health Board, whereby local women are recruited to support young single mothers, has worked well and is being adopted by other boards. A project to train Traveller women to advise Traveller families in relation to health issues has also proved successful. The development by health boards of family support services, including projects to help disadvantaged children, is further evidence of a commitment to go beyond the palliative and attack the causes of disadvantage and ill-health.[7]

These efforts are happening in parallel with those taking place under the national strategy to combat poverty, the partnership approach to local development and the county enterprise initiatives. Part of the problem is that so much is happening in parallel, rather than in a co-ordinated and planned attack on disadvantage and inequality. Nobody has overall responsibility in relation to tackling poverty and disadvantage in particular communities or areas, so it is not clear who is ensuring a co-ordinated approach. If such a framework existed, the impact of the work of the different agencies would likely be greater than the sum of the parts. Without it, the danger of duplication and turf battles is ever present.

The health services will continue to contribute to the economic and social development of the country in the next century. They have a particular contribution to make to reducing the health problems that disadvantaged individuals and communities face and to supporting parents with young children. This contribution will, however, be most effective within a framework of action by public bodies to tackle the economic and social causes of poverty.

---

[7] ibid. See pages 18–21 for examples of health board initiatives to tackle inequality and disadvantage.

INCREASING DEMOCRACY, OPENNESS AND TRANSPARENCY

As part of the democratic structure under which this country is governed, the health services have a responsibility to enhance the democratic process and to deepen the process in every walk of life. There are reasons for concern about the health of our democracy. Falling turnouts in elections, declining membership of political parties, difficulties in finding candidates to stand for public office and a widening gulf between the "ordinary" citizens and the political class are symptoms of a loss of confidence in our institutions that should not be ignored.[8]

The process of democratic accountability at national level has deepened in recent years with the expansion of the committee system of the Oireachtas, the greater involvement of members of committees in legislation and the increased opportunities for deputies and senators to hold ministers and their civil servants to account. Changes in the Comptroller and Auditor General Acts — whereby the C & AG audits the accounts of health boards and the chief executive officers are required to account to the committee of Public Accounts for the funds voted by the Oireachtas — have also increased the role of the Oireachtas in the monitoring of expenditure the health services. The Freedom of Information Act, 1997, changes the relationship between citizens and the institutions that govern them by giving the public a right to information held by a public body, both personal and of a policy nature. The extent to which the Act is used by citizens to hold public bodies and government accountable, as distinct from accessing information of interest to themselves, will be one of the most interesting issues that will arise as the Act is implemented.

Although health boards have a majority of elected representatives and are subject to the same standards of accountability as any publicly elected body, the lack of a well-developed regional level of government, the relative remoteness of the regional level from most of the issues affecting people in the health services and the fact that the

---

[8] Prof. Peter Mair, lecture to mark the 25th Anniversary of the MA in Politics Programme, Dublin Castle, 26 February 1998, reported in *The Irish Times*, 27 February 1998.

public representatives on health boards are indirectly elected, reduce the democratic profile of the boards. That said, the boards are the most well-developed democratic institutions we have at regional level and in a democratic society, their role deserves to be enhanced rather than reduced — as recommended, for example, by the Commission on Health Funding (*Report of the Commission on Health Funding*, 1989). It is

> the principle of direct election that gives local government (as distinct from local administration of miscellaneous services) a special degree of legitimacy and elected councillors their own special standing as legitimate spokespersons for the interests of those who elected them (*Towards a New Democracy — Implications for Local Government Reform*, 1985).

As with politics, most health services are local. The majority of health services can be managed and organised at the county level, or if a county is particularly small, between two counties. A regional structure is needed to deal with the large acute hospitals serving a regional catchment area and to ensure the coherent development of health services in the region as a whole. But there is scope for more democratic involvement at the county level in the organisation and delivery of services. How this could be done is a matter for debate, perhaps through a more structured relationship with the county and county borough councils. This relationship is needed anyway, as argued above, if the health service is to play its part in resolving the problems of disadvantaged communities.

The deepening of democracy is also about finding ways of encouraging the participation of an increasingly educated and sophisticated citizenry in the decisions that affect them. Such involvement is also critical to the health services mobilising the public for greater health and social gain. Greater involvement must be encouraged in a way that does not undermine the role of elected representatives or foster decision-making by the most organised and articulate interest group. The best example of a recent effort by the health boards at greater participation was the consultation they carried out with women in the preparation of the Plan for Women's Health. The women's movement had been very critical of many aspects of the health services as they affected women and of the unwillingness of health bodies and professionals to take their concerns on board. In 1995, in response to these criticisms, the Minister published the Discussion Document on Women's Health and asked each board to consult with women on the contents of the document (Department of Health, 1995). Each board, faced with the task of asking women what they thought of the health services and what they wanted from them, organised an innovative process of consultation with the assistance of member organisations of the National Women's Council of Ireland. Thousands of women were given an opportunity to make their views known through workshops, seminars, listening meetings and by post. In response to the views expressed by the women consulted and in the light of the *Plan for Women's Health*, published by the Department of Health in 1997, the management of each board has prepared or is preparing a regional plan to improve health services for women for adoption by the health board (Department of Health, 1997a). Each board has also established an advisory committee on women's health to ensure that the dialogue with women continues. While it is too soon to judge the impact of this process, it is clear that health boards now have a much better understanding of what women need from the health services and many women have been given an opportunity to influence the policy and operations of the health boards. The process has enhanced the democratic profile of the boards. There is no reason why a similar process should not work as well with other groups such as older people, people with disabilities, Travellers and people living in disadvantaged communities. It is important, however, that the boards take the lead role in this process of greater engagement with its citizens, who are also its consumers, as the statutory and democratically accountable body responsible for the health services.

ACHIEVING BETTER GOVERNMENT

As an important field of government activity, the health sector is also expected to contribute to the goal of achieving more effective and efficient government. More staff are employed in the health services than in any other public service and no other service employs so many registered professionals. With an estimated current expenditure of £2.78 billion in 1998 coming from the taxpayer, the health services are major consumers of public funds and have a responsibility to demonstrate that this funding is well spent.

The publication of the Health Strategy in 1994 — *Shaping a Healthier Future* — was a major step in ensuring the better governance of the health services. The Strategy provided a set of common objectives for the services — equity, quality and accountability — set out the changes in structures and relationships that were proposed to achieve these objectives and outlined a four-year plan to improve the health and personal social services. Four years on, a remarkable amount of what was set out in the Health Strategy has been achieved or is in train and, just as importantly, there are the beginnings of a common language and understanding of the problems affecting the health services and of the way to resolve them. It is fortunate that the four-year period of the Strategy coincided with an unprecedented expansion of the economy that meant resources were available to improve and develop the health services. However, the Health Strategy helped to ensure that the development happened in a planned and co-ordinated way. The Health Strategy has also helped to ensure that the health sector is responding to the Government's Strategic Management Initiative to manage the public service better and to make it more responsive to the people it serves.

The value of the Health Strategy has been proven and a continuation of the approach enshrined in that document is of great importance (O'Dwyer, 1997). A new strategy is being prepared to guide the health services in the first decade of the new millennium. On the basis of the issues raised in this chapter, the new strategy will have to give particular attention to co-ordination for health at national, regional and local level, the deepening of the democratic input to decision-making in the health services, and to the contribution the health services can play in achieving peace on this island.

ATTAINING PEACE ON THE ISLAND

One of the most exciting challenges facing the health services in the next few years will, hopefully, be the creation of opportunities to build peace on this island. The health services, both north and south, have a distinguished record of co-operation on issues of mutual interest. Ministers meet on a regular basis, civil servants share experiences and the health boards on both sides of the border have worked together for a number of years under the acronym CAWT — Co-operation and Working Together — and have secured funding from the European Union for this purpose. A most visible sign of co-operation will be the Institute of Public Health that is being established on a north/south basis. There is so much that is common in the two jurisdictions in relation to the philosophy and organisation of care, despite organisational changes in the north that have not been replicated in the south and a different approach to private practice in the south that is not shared in the north. There are also important bodies in the health services such as the Royal College of Physicians and the Royal College of Surgeons in Ireland that predate the division of the island and that have maintained their all-island identity. They will provide a useful model on which to build closer links across the health services, north and south.

Despite this level of co-operation, there is still much more that could be done if there were a framework in which one could look at the health needs of the population north and south as an entity, perhaps as part of a ministerial council with a health mandate. There is scope for building on common interests and formalising the arrangements that are in place already at ministerial and departmental level to foster a common approach to certain issues facing both systems. These issues include ensuring the best use of health resources for the population living close to the border, manpower planning, the assessment of new technology, the problem of waste disposal, and the ethical challenges posed by the advances in science and technology. It may take longer before some of the deeper differences in the two systems, such as the entitlements of the two populations to health services, can be tackled. But the aim should be to render the border increasingly insignificant in relation to access to health services and in the achievement of better health in all parts of the island. In particular, nothing should be done in the meantime that would increase the significance of the border as a barrier to accessing health and personal social services.

One of the differences between the two systems at present is the extent to which the Department of Health and Children is involved in European Union and World Health Organisation activities in the health field, and the extent to which the Department of Health and Social Services in the North is not. It would be of benefit to both parts of the island if arrangements could be made to ensure greater involvement by officials from the north in the main international forums concerned with health. There is no doubt of the support of both the EU and the WHO to assist in achieving peace on the island.

CONCLUSION

It is likely that, in the future, the health services will not be able to achieve their goals without the assistance of others, and other public bodies will not be able to achieve their goals without the assistance of the health services. If this assertion is true, it will have significant implications for the political and legislative framework in which the health services operate. The lead role of the health services in achieving health and social gain must be given greater recognition politically and in legislation, at the national, regional and local level.

On the other hand, the health services have a great deal to offer in attaining the national goals of economic and social development, the deepening of our democracy, the achievement of better government and the attainment of peace on the island. This contribution could be strengthened by a number of "framework" changes to rationalise the organisation of government activities, particularly at regional and county level, to ensure co-ordination in tackling the problems of disadvantaged communities, to increase participation in decision-making by citizens and to enable those involved in health services, north and south, to build on their shared interests. While the challenge to the political and legislative framework of the health services on the brink of the new millennium may seem daunting, it is one that our predecessors at the beginning of this century, faced with an apparently unconquerable toll of mortality and morbidity, might have envied.

References

Barrington, R. (1987), *Health, Medicine and Politics in Ireland 1900–1970*, Dublin: IPA.

Department of Finance (1998), "Estimates for Public Services (Abridged Version)", Dublin: Stationery Office.

Department of Health (1994), *Shaping a Healthier Future — A Strategy for Effective Health Care in the 1990s*, Dublin: Stationery Office.

Department of Health (1995a), *A Health Promotion Strategy*, Dublin: Stationery Office.

Department of Health (1995b), *Developing a Policy on Women's Health*, Dublin: Stationery Office.

Department of Health and Children (1996), "Health Service Personnel Census", 31 December, Dublin: Stationery Office.

Department of Health and Children (1997a), *A Plan for Women's Health*, Dublin: Stationery Office.

Department of Health and Children (1997b), *Enhancing the Partnership*, Dublin: Stationery Office.

Health Education Bureau (1987), *Promoting Health through Public Policy*, Dublin: HEB.

O'Dwyer, J. (1997), "Strategic Planning in the Irish Health Services", in *Reflections on Health — Commemorating Fifty Years of the Department of Health 1947–1997*, Dublin: IPA.

OECD (1997), *Economic Survey: Ireland*, Paris: OECD.

Report of the Commission on Health Funding (1989), Dublin: Stationery Office.

Towards a New Democracy — Implications for Local Government Reform (1985), Dublin: IPA.

WHO (1984), *Targets for Health for All*, Geneva: WHO

WHO (1997), *Investing in Health Research and Development*, Geneva: WHO.

WHO (forthcoming), *Health for All for the 21st Century*, Geneva: WHO.

Wiley, M. (1997), "Financing the Irish Health Services" in *Reflections on Health — Commemorating Fifty Years of the Department of Health 1947–1997*, Dublin: IPA.

PART TWO

Quality Management

6

MOVING TO A QUALITY CULTURE

Austin L. Leahy

INTRODUCTION

Fifty years ago, health care policy was largely dictated by doctors, nurses and other professionals, with management largely supplying administrative support. Patients' needs were addressed in a paternalistic manner, by and large. In the second half of the 20th century, the management view, and to a lesser extent the patients' view, were increasingly addressed in policy development. Publication of the Department of Health's strategy document, *Shaping a Healthier Future*, underlines the need for the views of the professional, the manager and the customer to be considered.

In the next century, the health care industry will become quality-driven. There will be increasing transparency and accountability, which will go far beyond our current expectations. These will operate at hospital level, at department level and also at individual level. Quality initiatives, which have largely been sporadic and individually driven in the 1990s, will need to be inculcated into the health system with a consequent development of a quality culture. At every level, this culture will require validation in the form of accreditation.

QUALITY IN THE 1990S

The post-industrial world has required an increasing dialogue between the producer and the users of a service. The health care industry has taken this on board by recognising that there are three views of quality that must be taken into account:

- The doctor's, nurse's, or other professional's view

- The manager's view, including that of the administrator, civil servant and politician

- The patient's view and that of their relatives.

Within health care, quality has been defined as doing the right thing consistently to ensure the best possible clinical outcome for patients, satisfaction for all customers, retention of talented staff and a good financial performance. In the 1990s, a number of successful experiments were undertaken which helped to define what the "right thing" was. Many of these initiatives were translated into practice through the establishment of standards. These were very helpful; however, they failed to become widely applied.

MOVEMENT TOWARDS A QUALITY CULTURE

In the 1980s and 1990s, it was increasingly recognised that quality must be considered under a number of headings. Robert Maxwell of the King's Fund has defined six:

1. Effectiveness or technical competence, which is an area often emphasised by the doctor;

2. Social acceptability, which is of particular concern to the patients and their relatives;

3. Efficiency, or the ability to deliver a service for the lowest unit cost;

4. Accessibility, which defines the availability of a service to the individual;

5. Relevance, which indicates that the service is that which is required by the individual and/or society;

6. Equity, indicating the equality of access to services. (*Journal of the Irish Colleges of Physicians and Surgeons*, Vol. 26, No. 2, April 1997)

Services in the Irish health system were increasingly evaluated by these parameters. Instead of providing a number of ill-defined services, albeit while guaranteeing their technical competence, health care providers increasingly had to address other aspects of quality. The Hospital In-Patient Enquiry (HIPE), which was initiated in the 1980s in all acute sector hospitals, was given additional impetus in the 1990s. The financial allocations of acute sector hospitals were adjusted on the basis of their recorded output on the HIPE. For the first time, this allowed estimates of activity and complexity to be used in the Irish health system.

The waiting list initiative was a further example of efficiency measures being introduced. In this instance, certain services with long waiting lists were singled out for increased provision, with hospitals being remunerated by additional funding. Driven by the Department of Health, this initiative underlined the importance of accessibility and relevance. There were many, many other examples of centrally driven quality initiatives, all of which served to indicate the direction of government policy.

In a more bottom-up approach, individuals became involved in quality initiatives right across the health system. This was exemplified by the formation of organisations dedicated to the pursuit of quality within the Irish health care system, such as the Irish Society for Quality in Health Care, which was established in 1994. This approach was particularly welcome because it was multidisciplinary and was occurring at all levels of the health system. Professional organisations such as the Royal College of Surgeons in Ireland also emphasised the need for a quality approach, even beyond service provision, to encompass professional training and ongoing accreditation.

The movement towards a widespread quality culture in the Irish health care system is compelling and irreversible. It will ensure that health outcomes are improved, and will do so while attempting to control expenditure and to limit waste. Within the new order, accountability is no longer optional. In the 21st century, it will be increasingly demanded by politicians, the Department of Health and patients or patients' organisations. Strategies will be defined which ensure that quality is both delivered and seen to be delivered. This movement is likely to escalate as expectations are defined more clearly.

In the current system, the patients' expectations are rarely expressed and seldom debated, and consequently lead to escalating litigation. Many of the frustrations in the health system emanate from a lack of clarity concerning expectations. Once these expectations are defined and adjusted by what can be realistically provided, then an explicit contract can be drawn up. The term "rationing" has been used for the process whereby patients' reasonable expectations are defined. Once these have been defined in a dialogue between the professional, the manager and the patient, they can lead to attempts to maximise all parameters of quality. This can only encourage health care professionals, as standards can be continuously enforced and improved.

OVERCOMING RESISTANCE TO QUALITY

It would be naive to propose that the development of a quality culture in the 21st century will be universally supported. Resistance will occur at the individual level by professionals, managers and patients. Professionals have a genuine feeling that the health system is different and that the complexity of the environment and of outcomes make measurement difficult. Furthermore, quality initiatives are seen to challenge the coping mechanisms required by professionals to survive in the stressful environment of our health system. Managers may be unclear about the advantage of broadening the quality debate. Financial considerations and political expediencies may inhibit discussion on priorities within the health services.

The debate which must take place to deliver a quality culture may confuse and antagonise the patient and patient advocacy organisations. Any attempt at clarifying expectations will be seen as an attempt to impose rationing. This will of necessity require a statesmanlike approach by our politicians.

Dialogue will be the cornerstone of the development of a quality culture. In managing this evolution, strategies must be designed to address individual and organisational resistance. Altering the culture of hospitals into one which accepts the needs to improve processes in a non-threatening environment will require vision by all concerned. It will require professionals to relinquish power that is currently being exercised unilaterally, thereby allowing a multi-disciplinary approach.

Quality initiatives will need to be promoted both nationally and at an organisational level. Instruments will have to be developed centrally that will impose realistic performance indicators based on what standards can be provided within existing resources. The next century will see the development of a twin strategy approach to quality. There will also be an initiation of continuous quality improvement (CQI), leading to multidisciplinary teams refining health care processes. There will be an establishment of accountability through quality assurance.

CONTINUOUS QUALITY IMPROVEMENT

The next century will see an immersion of health care organisations in a quality culture. This emphasis on continuous quality improvement (CQI) will ensure that every area of all health care organisations will be subjected to quality improvement. There will be a system-wide and comprehensive strategy within all organisations aimed at raising the standards of patient care through improving all work processes.

During the second half of the 20th century, CQI became a developing influence within manufacturing and service industries worldwide. Its expansion within the health care industry in the next century will lead to a reduction in the variation of task performance, with processes being more consistently defined. This will result in an improvement in patient care and an empowering of all employees involved in care delivery.

By reducing the necessary variation or unpredictability in processes, and by continually attempting to improve standards, CQI will improve care for all patients. It has, therefore, got a wide and systemic impact on quality of care. A multidisciplinary approach is central to the development of CQI. Previously, most quality programmes were promoted by single disciplines, as exemplified by clinical audit. This neglects to emphasise the diversity of disciplines involved in each process of care. Furthermore, the complexity of outcomes also makes a more multidisciplinary approach desirable.

A number of elements will be required to ensure that a quality culture succeeds. At the outset, there must be a commitment from the top. This not only implies that the political will exists to develop a culture based on quality, but also that leaders of all disciplines within the health system must empower their departments and workers. Such a devolution of power will only be achieved by considerable effort and perseverance.

In tandem with the empowerment of all departments and workers throughout the health care organisation, there will be provision of adequate resources for each voice to be heard. Employees can be organised in quality improvement teams, each working to tackle specific problems and processes. Communications will be central to CQI, with workers and teams connected through regular meetings, both in person and through the facility of information technology.

At the outset, there must be a clear idea of customer priorities. As well as assessing customer expectations, the patient's perception of quality of care delivered must be continuously monitored.

A number of studies have been carried out to clarify patient's view of quality. In the 21st century, it will be important that these opportunities are provided throughout the system and continuously. It is proposed that a complete picture of patient's requirements will result and patient's expectations will be adequately addressed. Once patient expectations are translated into priorities, processes and systems aimed at meeting these expectations can be designed. Advances in information technology will allow these strategies to be implemented consistently.

Above all, the culture of the organisation will need to be supportive of CQI. Our current organisational structure will need to be adapted so that we develop a "seamless" organisation. In the Irish health care system, moving from a top-down approach will require a huge amount of personal effort by managers and professionals. Natural caution about relinquishing power must give way to communication, trust and empowerment. This will go hand-in-glove with the development of incentives for organisations and individuals to move to a quality approach. The contribution of the individual and various teams will be acknowledged using financial and other incentives.

Inevitably, the processes chosen for examination will be prioritised by the professional, the manager and the patient in a CQI approach. While we must concentrate on the patients' expectations, it is also important that these expectations are clarified in the event that they are unrealistic. A number of clinical protocols could be developed where multidisciplinary teams would examine the systems. This could be as simple as the management of pain, bedsores or specific conditions such as strokes. Violations of admission procedures, discharge procedures, or clinical protocols leading to changes in patient management could be used as an index of the health of the organisation. Certain departments, such as the Accident & Emergency Department, Records Department, Catering, Information Technology and Patient Services, would easily lend themselves to examination. Communications and complaints are other areas that might be examined. By establishing quality circles of professionals to examine these processes and produce improvements, multifactorial outcomes related to these processes can be identified. This will allow a reduction in the variance of patient care, reduce waste and focus on patient needs.

QUALITY ASSURANCE

Quality assurance involves defining acceptable standards and detecting processes that lie outside these standards. By examining these exceptions, we can better understand our processes and avoid unpredictability in the future. If CQI involves the reduction of variation in all processes, then quality assurance involves detecting those processes that lie outside acceptable standards. In the next century, quality assurance will be implemented throughout the health system.

There will be centralised definition of acceptable standards, each applicable to the various areas of the health services. At a local level, their implementation will be supervised by quality assurance departments. All workers will be involved in continuous quality assurance by detecting processes that lie outside acceptable standards and examining these in formal meetings and informally through communication.

By consistently assessing the quality of care delivered and comparing it with agreed standards, quality can be reinforced in a transparent way. If deficiencies are perceived, then either the standards are unattainable, which requires an examination of resources or expectations, or else the processes are flawed and need to be revised.

Development of HIPE and other administrative support structures for bed management, communications, etc., will be centralised in quality assurance departments. The department will report to the clinical and management structures but will essentially be responsive to patient demand and have a direct relationship with the Department of Health. Where changes are indicated in the pursuit of quality, the quality assurance department will be responsible to ensure that the health care organisation meets these demands. In assisting the organisation to achieve these changes, a process of accreditation will be introduced throughout the health system, which will lead to support being exchanged by organisations.

ACCREDITATION — A STRATEGY FOR QUALITY IN IRELAND IN THE 21ST CENTURY

If the health system is to respond to democratic needs and deliver a quality culture, this will need to be actively managed. In the past, a number of enthusiasts have championed quality within the health services. This individual effort needs to be promoted, formalised, and disseminated. This can be achieved through accreditation. The Department of Health will implement health service accreditation by defining standards which identify both minimum safe service provision and also examples of best practice. At a national level, these standards will be produced through wide consultation and testing in the field. From this, accreditation instruments will be generated. These are practical tools which confirm that a standard is being adequately achieved.

All workers in the health system would be expected to participate in conducting internal self-assessment. There will also be external assessment designed to confirm a uniformity of care to patients. For the Department of Health, the process of accreditation is attractive, as it leads to improved patient care, an active risk management strategy and independent recognition of conformity.

CONCLUSIONS

In the 21st century, the Irish health system will have a quality culture which will involve continuing debate and compromise between various stakeholders, and empowerment of individuals. The variations which are tolerated in the 1990s will be addressed by CQI and quality assurance programmes. At a national level, the Department of Health will recognise these needs by resourcing an accreditation programme and supporting individuals and teams who are involved in a CQI approach.

This programme will develop directly from clinical audit programmes, quality assurance programmes and individual quality initiatives which previously were random in their approach. Developments in communications and alterations in the structure of the health services will underpin this approach.

There will be increasing specification with regards to patient expectation. Processes which began in the 1980s, referred to as rationing, will be refined in the next century. Contracts will be made directly with patients, ensuring delivery of quality care. Through its central accreditation process, the Department of Health will ensure that quality is maintained and patients can be guaranteed a uniformity of care throughout the health services.

7

RISK MANAGEMENT AS A STRATEGY FOR QUALITY

Denis Cusack

HEALTH CARE RISK MANAGEMENT

As we approach the 21st century, there is a proper and pertinent emphasis on quality in health care. However, although we live in an age of increasing consumerism with an eye to delivery of quality service to the consumer, it would be wrong to view this as a new concept in the health care setting. The very essence of the carer–patient relationship is one of trust where the health carer strives to deliver and the patient expects to receive a high quality of care. At the end of the 17th century, one of the fundamental objectives of the College of Physicians was set out as follows:

> For the encouragement of the learned and experienced practitioners in physic and for the benefit of (the King's) good subjects.[1]

The 1994 Government health strategy is underpinned by the key principles of equity, quality of service and accountability (Department of Health, 1994).

The modern concept of risk management arose in the industrial area in the Far East in the 1960s and 1970s and was adopted by the American health care industry in the 1980s in the face of an increasing medical litigation crisis. However, a much broader view must be taken of health care risk management. It is a critical tool in the im-

---

[1] The Charter of the Royal College of Physicians of Ireland (1692), line 7.

provement of health care delivery and is intrinsic to any strategy for quality. Too often it is seen merely as an answer to the economic downside of the medical litigation crisis. It is true that it will have the effect of decreasing litigation and it has been said that for every pound put into risk management, four pounds will be returned in the long term by decreased costs. However, this should not be the driving force to the introduction of health care risk management. By decreasing risks to patients and staff, quality will be improved. Important examples are in the area of risk to patients from less-than-optimum standard of care, and in the areas of clinical records, consent and drug administration.

Health care risk management is only one component of an overall solution. However, it is the only one which takes a proactive and preventive approach with the primary aim of improving quality of health care delivery.

Unfortunately, there has not been a full and proper commitment from many of the health care institutions in the area of risk management. Too often this has been left to interested health carers on an *ad hoc* basis. They have been poorly equipped, poorly staffed, poorly paid and have been provided with poor facilities. Too often, it has been left to middle management or nursing management without a proper input from senior management and hospital consultants.

Unless there is a proper commitment to the introduction of health care risk management, it will not succeed. This requires commitment from hospital consultants, health care administrators and the Department of Health.

Health care risk management will only succeed as a strategy for health care quality if it is fully understood by these various people. This chapter aims to assist in this understanding of risk management as applied to health care delivery and quality.

MEDICAL LITIGATION: CRISIS?

There has been a significant increase in the incidence of negligence claims taken by patients against hospitals, doctors, nurses and health care professionals in general in the past 20 years. There has also been a significant increase in the number of actions taken by employees against their employers in relation to injuries at work. It is in the context of this litigation crisis that the process of risk management is most frequently mentioned. This process is one whereby risks to the patient, employees and other persons are identified and anticipated and measures put in place to eliminate, avoid or minimise those risks. As stated, health care risk management was initiated as an active process in the United States in the mid-1980s following the recognition of the medical malpractice crisis which was costing the US one billion dollars by 1985 (Scheid, 1998). The direct cost of medical indemnity to the Irish State in 1998 is £25 million but the indirect costs are several times this figure.

In both the clinical and non-clinical health care settings, risk will always exist. Risk may be viewed as the possibility of an adverse occurrence leading to legal claims and other losses. Although medical litigation is often said to cost an arm and a leg, the Code of Hammurabi, *circa* 2000 BC, stated:

> If a physician operates on a man for a severe wound with a bronze lancet and causes a man's death, or opens an abscess in the eye of a man with a bronze lancet and destroys the man's eye, they shall cut off his fingers.

Thankfully such a penalty does not exist in the Irish legal code today.

No single approach will resolve this litigation crisis. Health care risk management is truly only one component of an overall possible solution with a number of elements:

- Health care Risk Management
- Mediation
- Arbitration
- Pre-trial Screening
- No Fault Compensation
- Structured Settlements
- Capping of Awards

- Statutory Early Offers
- Early Exchange of Medical Reports
- Handling of Small Claims (Woolf Report).

Many people mistakenly view the role of health care risk management as being solely the reduction in incidence and cost of medical litigation. However, its primary function is an improvement in the delivery of quality health care to the patient and of a quality health care environment to employees and others in the health care sector. Nevertheless, legitimate questions have been raised about the necessity for risk management and whether it is a realistic expectation that it would reduce the litigation bill (Dingwall and Fenn, 1991).

In the much-quoted Harvard study, 3.7 per cent of hospital admissions involved an adverse event. These included: death, readmission after discharge, fever and unplanned transfer to ITU. In one per cent of admissions, the care delivered was judged to be negligent (Hiatt et al., 1989; for the detailed results of the study, see Brennan et al., 1991; Leape et al., 1991; and Localio et al., 1991). Applying the Harvard figures to an Irish hospital with 20,000 admissions per annum, one would expect 740 adverse events, 30 deaths and 15 cases of permanent disability per annum due to an adverse event. In the Harvard study, one out of seven incidents proceeded to a legal claim. However, it is not only the financial cost but also the non-financial cost to patient and staff that must be considered. Risk management must be an integral component of health care practice: clinical, non-clinical and administrative. It is, however, a relatively new concept in Ireland (Cusack, 1994).

THE HEALTH CARE RISK MANAGEMENT PROCESS

Health care risk management is a process that identifies accidents or other untoward incidents which put a patient's or employee's health or safety at risk. It aims to eliminate or reduce those risks, leading to an improvement in patient health care and the health care working environment. It also aims to reduce litigation claims and also the harmful financial and other effects of a claim, once initiated.

It is therefore a preventative and treatment process and it has five basic elements, as follows:

- Risk Identification

- Risk Analysis

- Risk Treatment

- Risk Evaluation

- Claims Management.

The risk management process thus aims to reduce harm and improve care, but it also recognises the ever-present element in risk that can never be wholly eliminated — the human factor (Reason, 1995). The prerequisites for effective health care risk management are proper financial, personnel and structural foundations.

RISK IDENTIFICATION AND ANALYSIS

The first step in the process must be to identify the risks. This can be done by a number of methods. The most traditional of these is the incident report. However, this can be made more effective by being expanded to include any "near misses". Thus any adverse occurrence, whether or not it has caused injury or harm, is identified. It would also be possible to identify a particular area of risk or a particular procedure which is known to entail risk and to identify any adverse occurrences in this specific way over a specified period of time. Use of reports from the patient services office, the Chaplaincy services, infection control units, clinical audit, patients' complaints procedures and external consultancy audits could also be used, in any combination, as a source of reports. Medical audit could also be incorporated into risk identification and it shares with risk management the primary aim of maintaining or improving the standard of patient care. Such a process includes clear definition of a systematic review of clinical outcome and the use of comparative data as a "benchmark" from which standards of care can be improved (Leahy et al., 1996).

The use of clinical indicators contributes to the identification of significant trends in clinical practice that may expose patients to risk of injury (MMI Companies Inc., 1993). Such clinical risk or warning indicators include:

- Unexpected death

- New neurological deficit

- Unplanned return to the operating theatre

- Unplanned admission to ITU

- Adverse medication problem

- Failure to act on a laboratory report

- Equipment malfunction

- Mislaid clinical records.

Once a risk has been identified, it must be analysed before it can be managed. This can be done quite simply according to potential claim cost, frequency of occurrence of adverse incident and cost of measures to manage such incidents. In essence, what is being measured and analysed is the potential severity of something going wrong. This part of the process can also analyse why things go wrong. Thus, in anaesthetics it may be a failure to check equipment and unfamiliarity with the equipment; in obstetrics, it may be inadequate foetal monitoring, mismanagement of forceps or lack of senior staff involvement in delivery. Adverse incidents are rarely the result of a single error and usually point to a collection of deficiencies in the health care delivery. Very often, this is a series of errors with unusual circumstances.

RISK CONTROL AND CLAIMS MANAGEMENT

Having identified and analysed the risk, the next part of the process is to avoid, eliminate or reduce, or transfer the risk. Review of the standards of care, clinical guidelines and protocols are all part of risk control in the clinical setting (see below). In the non-clinical sphere, the implementation of the statutory requirements of the safety at work legislation exemplifies the risk management process (see below). In relation to the funding of potential negligence claims, three major methods have been recognised: pay as you go; funding for reported liabilities (claims-made basis); or funding for all liability (claims-occurred basis). One of the difficulties facing health care administrators and insurers is the typical delay between incidence occurrence and reporting of a potential claim and the further delay before any due payment is made. This is known as the "scorpion effect" — the sting in the tail.

The entire risk management process must be constantly reviewed and evaluated to ensure that it is effective and achieving its aim of improving health care and the health care working environment.

Risk control also involves management of any claim relating to an incident which has occurred. Central to this, and an appropriate approach in improving health care delivery, must be the existence of an accessible and workable complaints procedure.

CLINICAL AND NON-CLINICAL RISK MANAGEMENT IN ACTION

One of the first examples of clinical audit forming part of an early risk management process on this side of the Atlantic was the national Confidential Enquiry into Perioperative Deaths (CEPOD) carried out in Britain in the 1980s. One of the aims of CEPOD was to attempt to determine mortality rates associated with surgical procedures up to 30 days after the procedure had been carried out. CEPOD was thus about the quality of health care delivery and the equity of health care standards across Britain (Buck et al., 1987). A second such study resulted in the Report on Confidential Enquiries into Maternal Deaths (CEMD) in the UK for the period 1991–93 (Hibbard et al., 1996). Similar studies, as part of an overall risk management policy, could be used beneficially to improve health care delivery and quality in Ireland in the 21st century.

In the non-clinical area, it must be recognised that the provision of ancillary and support services is an intrinsic part of health care delivery to patients. Inherent in this, however, are risks to patients, to visitors, to health care institutions and to employees. In 1996, the Irish Insurance Federation noted that, in the area of employer's liability, there had been an 18 per cent increase in net incurred claims, to a total of £129.5 million. According to the Health and Safety Authority, 4,500 accidents were reported to the Authority in 1996 and it is generally believed that this is a significant under-representation of the total number of accidents at work (Health and Safety Authority, 1996). The Safety, Health and Welfare at Work Act, 1989, and all of the Regulations from European Union sources and Irish domestic legislative sources, are perhaps the finest pieces of public health legislation enacted throughout Europe in the 20th century. They will only come to fruition in the 21st century. As a strategy for improvement in safety and health at work and in health care delivery, an understanding of the major pieces of legislation in this area is essential.[2] Indeed, the general principles of prevention set out in the first schedule of the 1993 Regulations are an excellent example of practical risk management. They are as follows:

a) The avoidance of risks.

b) The evaluation of unavoidable risks.

c) The combating of risks at source.

d) The adaptation of work to the individual, especially as regards the design of places of work, the choice of work equipment and the choice of systems of work, with a view, in particular to alleviating monotonous work and work at a predetermined workrate and to reducing their effect on health.

e) The adaptation of the place of work to technical progress.

f) The replacement of dangerous articles, substances or systems at work by non-dangerous or less dangerous articles, substances or systems.

---

[2] See, for example, Sections 6 and 12 (1) of the Safety, Health and Welfare at Work Act, 1989, and paragraphs 5, 10, 11 and 13 of the Safety Health and Welfare at Work (General Applications) Regulations, 1993.

g) The development of an adequate prevention policy in relation to safety, health and welfare at work, which takes account of technology, organisation of work, working conditions, social factors and the influence of factors related to the working environment.

h) The giving to collective protective measures of priority over individual protective measures.

i) The giving of appropriate training and instructions to employees.

CLINICAL RISK MANAGEMENT

Lest it be forgotten in this review of risk management as a strategy to improve health care delivery, at the core of such a service is, of course, *clinical care*. Indeed, both the professional standard and the legal standard of care are central to understanding quality of patient care. There is no evidence that the standards of professional training or skill have fallen. Nevertheless, the ever-increasing amount of knowledge which every health carer must acquire, together with the ever-increasing complexity of technology and the greater expectation of patients in relation to health care delivery, have led to a serious crisis of confidence in this sphere. It is here that risk management can be most effectively used as a tool in improving patient care in the 21st century.

Under Irish law, the standard of care in relation to medical treatment which a doctor owes to a patient has been set out in the Dunne case:

> The true test for establishing negligence in diagnosis or treatment on the part of a medical practitioner is whether he has been proved to be guilty of such failure as no medical practitioner of equal specialist or general status and skill would be guilty of, if acting with ordinary care.[3]

This standard is determined by a judge sitting alone after hearing the facts and expert evidence. In that case, Chief Justice Finlay said that:

---

[3] Dunne (an infant) v National Maternity Hospital and Jackson [1989] *Irish Reports* 91.

General and approved practice need not be universal but must be approved of and adhered to by a substantial number of reputable practitioners holding the relevant specialist or general qualifications.

Expert testimony will not be conclusive, nor will the existence or adherence or otherwise to guidelines or protocols be conclusive one way or the other. Nevertheless, such guidelines or protocols may be introduced to a judge by an expert witness as evidence of accepted standards of care. However, guidelines as part of a clinical risk management process are only discretionary. They will certainly assist junior members of the health care team in dealing with common medical problems and in dealing with complex medical situations. They are only guidelines and should not be adhered to slavishly, but must always yield to reasonable clinical judgement. On the other hand, deviation from a guideline or protocol which results in patient injury would have to be justified.

Areas of patient care in which risk management can be of great value include the obtaining of informed consent and the maintenance of adequate and proper clinical records. These two areas are ones of concern and are frequently at issue in medical litigation.

Risk management can also assist in the introduction of a new procedure and quality assessment of same. A recent example is minimal access surgery. Certain procedures carried out in this way — in particular gynaecological procedures — resulted in an unacceptably high incidence of patient injury. Studies showed that this was due to trial-and-error learning, work overload, long shifts and reluctance to admit limitations during a training programme. Patient demand may also have had an influence on the too-ready acceptance of minimal access surgery because it caused less pain, had a shorter hospital stay, led to less scarring and a much quicker return to activity. A quality review carried out by the Royal Surgical Colleges of Great Britain and Ireland exemplifies the positive role for a risk management process in planning health care (Senate of the Royal Surgical Colleges of Great Britain and Ireland, 1994).

The risk management process can also look at specific events such as discharge from psychiatric care and the risk of suicide, the prescribing, dispensing and administration of drugs and wrong medication, and the non-follow-up of radiological reporting, resulting in missed fracture being examples. General practice, public health medicine, midwifery and nursing care are also amenable to risk management (Greene, 1997; Dineen, 1997; Berragan, 1994).

The setting-up of proper complaints procedures for patients to follow when a real or perceived difficulty arises is one aspect of risk management that could be very usefully applied as part of the strategy for the new century. Formal complaints procedures are not the norm in Irish health care systems to date. In the hospitals and health boards, procedures vary widely, both in form and effectiveness. Although a formal complaints procedure does exist in the general medical services, it is under-utilised and is certainly not comparable to the complaints procedures within the National Health Service general practice in Britain (Day, 1997). A risk management review of the standard of clinical care can be carried out in a number of ways. If funding allows, it should be applied on an institution-wide basis. If full funding is not available, clinical risk management can be applied in an ongoing way over a period of time taking specific areas, specialities, interventions or incidents, such as:

Clinical Specialities:

- Obstetrics

- Gynaecology

- Orthopaedics

- Anaesthetics

- Accident & Emergency

- General Surgery.

Specific Interventions:

- Laparoscopic Herniorraphy

- Perinatal Asphyxia

- Scaphoid X-Ray

- Anaesthetic Awareness
- Transthoracic Endoscopic Sympathectomy
- Diagnosis of Bacterial Meningitis.

Geographical Area:
- A & E Department
- Medical Records Department
- Operating Theatre
- Out-Patients' Department
- Delivery Suite
- Patient Services Office
- Pharmacy Department.

Geographical Area and Incident:
- A & E Department (Failure to X-Ray)
- Operating Theatre (Retained Instrument or Swab)
- Cleaning Services (Needlestick Injury)
- Out-Patients Department (Missing Chart)
- Delivery Suite (CTG Tracings)
- Patients' Services Office (Complaints Handling)
- Pharmacy Department (Incorrect labelling).

Problems Shared by all Departments:
- Communications
- Staff experience and training
- Consent
- Clinical Records
- Protocols.

Administrative procedures may also be amenable to review and would include such matters as the maintenance of specimen signatures of clinical staff, staff records and the tracing of previous employees.

Finally, in reviewing risk management as a strategy to improve health care, the input of patients should not be forgotten. The emergence of patient organisations such as the Irish Patients Association will hopefully be a positive step in a co-operative process between patients and their health carers in the next century. The patients' charter should also be viewed in this context, although it is aspirational rather than legally binding and must be viewed in the political context of its time (Department of Health, 1992).

ACHIEVING A SUCCESSFUL RISK MANAGEMENT PROCESS

If it is accepted that health care risk management forms part of the strategy for quality improvement in the Irish health system in the next century, then it is necessary for all health care institutions and organisations, be they large or small, to consider how best to achieve this. The human element in this cannot be underestimated and is best served by employing a person skilled in risk management and by risk management training for health care personnel in general. The risk manager is essential to the overall process and ideally should have training and experience in at least two of the following fields: clinical practice, law, medical litigation, administration and insurance. To date, there has been little more than tokenism and lack of co-operation in the training of risk management specialists. Large institutions must be prepared to fund such a post and the continuing education of the risk manager. For smaller institutions, it may not be feasible to have a full-time risk manager; a suitable compromise is to have a person in a part-time position, perhaps shared with another post, or to employ the services of a risk manager on a consultancy basis.

Even with the appointment of a risk manager, the process will not be successful if it is viewed as a position held by one person rather than as a process involving all carers (clinical and administrative), facilitated by the risk manager. Training of all health care personnel in the administrative, medical, nursing, other health care specialities and the non-clinical areas must be undertaken. In 1995, a post-graduate Higher Diploma in Health Care Risk Management was initiated by the Medical Faculty at University College Dublin in association with the Medical Protection Society and supported by the Department of Health. This is an example of the co-operative role of medical educators, medical indemnifiers and the Government, which is necessary to improve future health care quality. To date, some 70 health care professionals from all the specialities have received basic training in risk management on this course.

The founding of the Irish Association of Risk Management in March 1998 is a progressive step and it is hoped that it will develop and be an inclusive organisation for all of those with the relevant qualifications or expertise and a continuing interest in risk management. It is an unfortunate truth that the most active health care practitioners in risk management are often in the areas of nursing or administration. With a few notable exceptions, medical practitioners are rarely actively involved in risk management. All of these sectors must be involved for the process to succeed.

Each institution with a genuine interest in risk management must also set up a risk management committee. This must be multi-disciplinary and look not only at individual incidents but also assess patterns of incidents so that preventive measures can be put into place in accordance with organisational policy. The committee must also be the co-ordinator of educational programmes for staff, since this is an essential foundation stone for the process. For those larger institutions with a medical director, such a person would be an ideal bridge, together with the risk manager, between clinical and administrative areas.

Staff training must involve education in medico-legal concepts, such as informed consent and the keeping of clinical records. All health care professionals should be encouraged to train in health care management as part of the risk management process and accreditation processes for hospitals, and individuals must take cognisance of such training. Health care workers have initially been somewhat hostile to risk management, viewing it as a potential way to point the finger of blame at individuals and departments. Encouraging a positive attitude amongst staff towards clinical risk management and showing it to be a non-threatening supportive system for staff is the duty of management (O'Connor, 1996).

The government must also play a role in encouraging the positive contribution to be made by clinical risk management. This could be in the form of an incentive akin to a "no claims bonus", which rewards those institutions that have introduced effective risk management. Such a reward system is already in place in the UK for members of the Clinical Negligence Scheme for Trusts (CNST) (Hickey, 1995).

On occasion, the risk management process appears to fail. However, this is not usually a failure of the process itself but is due to a lack of systems, failure to follow up incidents, inexperienced and poorly trained staff, deficiencies in complaints handling, lack of resources or poor management commitment.

TOWARDS THE 21ST CENTURY — THE LARGER CONTEXT

Health care risk management has proven to be an effective tool in improving health care delivery to patients. The financial benefits will only be seen in the longer term. Risk management is only part of an overall process to improve the present situation, but should be seen as an end in itself to improve health care delivery and not merely as a means of limiting the effects of medical litigation. It is nonetheless one of the solutions to the present unacceptable medical litigation crisis. But it is a greater part of the way forward for improvement in quality of health care delivery in the 21st century, and it requires commitment in terms of personnel, resources and finances. It deserves more than tokenism. It must be an inherent part of the strategy for quality.

References

Berragan, L. (1994), "The Concept of Quality Care", *Journal of Community Nursing*, Vol. 8, No. 7, p. 36.

Brennan, T.A., L.L. Leape, N.M. Laird et al. (1991), "Incidence of Adverse Events and Negligence in Hospitalised Patients: Results of the Harvard Medical Practice Study I", *New England Journal of Medicine;* Vol. 324, No. 6, p. 370

Buck, N., H.B. Devlin, J.N. Lunn (1987), *Report of Confidential Enquiry into Perioperative Deaths (CEPOD)*, London: Nuffield Provincial Hospitals Trust/King's Fund.

Cusack, D. (1994), "Health Care Risk Management", *Journal of the Irish Colleges of Physicians and Surgeons*, Vol. 23, No. 3, p. 176.

Day, A.T. (1997), "General Practice and the New Complaints Procedures", *Clinical Risk*, Vol. 3, p. 132.

Department of Health (1992), *Patients' Charter*, Dublin: Stationery Office.

Department of Health (1994), *Shaping a Healthier Future: Strategy for Effective Health Care in the 1990s*, Dublin: Stationery Office.

Dineen, M. (1997), "Clinical Risk Management and Midwives", *Modern Midwife*, Vol. 7, No. 11, p. 9.

Dingwall, R. and P. Fenn (1991), "Is Risk Management Necessary?" *Journal of Risk Safety Medicine*, Vol. 2, p. 91.

Greene, S. (1997), "Clinical Risk and the General Practitioner", *Clinical Risk*, Vol. 3, p. 143.

Health and Safety Authority (1996), Annual Report, Dublin: HSA.

Hiatt, H.H., B.A. Barnes, T.A. Brennan, et al. (1989), "A Study of Medical Injury and Medical Malpractice: An Overview", *New England Journal of Medicine;* Vol. 321, No. 7, p. 480.

Hibbard, B.M., M.M. Anderson, J.O. Drife et al. (1996), *Report on Confidential Enquiries into Maternal Deaths in the UK 1991–1993.* London: HMSO.

Hickey, J. (1995), "The Clinical Negligence Scheme for Trusts: Risk Management — A New Approach", *Clinical Risk*, Vol. 1, p. 43.

Leahy, A.L., M. Sharkey, M. Wiley, et al. (1996), "Unit Based Surgical Audit: Measuring the Quality of Clinical Practice", *Journal of the Irish Colleges of Physicians and Surgeons*, Vol. 25, No. 1: 47.

Leape, L.L., T.A. Brennan, N.M. Laird et al. (1991), "The Nature of Adverse Events and Negligence in Hospitalised Patients: Results of the Harvard Medical Practice Study II", *New England Journal of Medicine;* Vol. 324, No. 6, p. 377.

Localio, A.R., A.G. Lawthers, T.A. Brennan et al. (1991), "Relation between Malpractice Claims and Adverse Events due to Negligence: Results of the Harvard

Medical Practice Study III", *New England Journal of Medicine*; Vol. 325, No. 4, p. 245;

MMI Companies Inc. (1993), "Clinical Risk Modification — An Eight Year Data Summary", Deerfield, IL: MMI Companies Inc.

O'Connor, A.M. (1996), "The Attitude of the Staff towards Clinical Risk Management", *Clinical Risk*, Vol. 2, p. 119.

Reason, J. (1995), "Understanding Adverse Events: Human Factors" Chapter 3 in C. Vincent, *Clinical Risk Management*, London: BMJ Publishing Group.

Scheid, J.H. (1998), "American Statutory Responses to the Medical Malpractice Crisis", *Medico-Legal Journal of Ireland*, Vol. 4, No. 1, p. 3.

Senate of the Royal Surgical Colleges of Great Britain and Ireland (1994), *Quality Assurance: The Role of Training, Certification, Audit and Continuing Professional Education in the Maintenance of the Highest Possible Standards of Surgical Practice*, London: Royal College of Surgeons of England.

8

QUALITY OF LIFE ASSESSMENT: AN IMPORTANT INDICATOR OF HEALTH GAIN

Ciaran A. O'Boyle

INTRODUCTION

The assessment of patients' quality of life is assuming increasing importance in medicine and health care (Spilker, 1990; 1996). In the UK, quality of life, health status and the experiences of patients and carers are explicitly identified as among the significant indicators of health gain (Department of Health (UK), 1992). The Irish Department of Health, in its strategy document *Shaping a Healthier Future* (1994), proposed that:

> The concepts of health gain and social gain, allied to greatly improved data collection and analysis, will be used to focus prevention, treatment and care more clearly on improvements in health status or quality of life.

The Department of Health's *Plan for Women's Health* for the years 1997–99 has four main objectives, one of which is to maximise the health and social gain of Irish women. The two principal objectives of the recent National Cancer Strategy (Department of Health, 1996) are: (i) to take all measures possible to reduce rates of illness and death from cancer and (ii) to ensure that those who develop cancer receive the most effective care and treatment and that their quality of life is enhanced to the greatest possible extent.

Figure 8.1: Definitions of Health Gain and Social Gain used in Shaping a Healthier Future *(Department of Health, 1994)*

Health gain is described as being concerned with health status, both in terms of increases in life expectancy and in terms of some improvements in the quality of life through the cure or alleviation of an illness or disability or through any other general improvement in the health of the individual or the population at whom the service is directed.

Social gain is concerned with broader aspects of the quality of life. It includes, for example, the quality added to the lives of dependent elderly people and their carers as a result of the provision of support services, or the benefit to a child of living in an environment free from physical or psychological abuse.

The terms health gain and social gain as used in these documents both make reference to quality of life (Figure 8.1) and are used to indicate that patients and clients of the health or personal social services should receive a clear benefit from their contact with the system. These terms have also found their way into the Department of Health's mission statement, which includes the aspiration:

> to protect, promote and restore the health and well-being of people by ensuring that health and social services are planned, managed and delivered to achieve measurable health and social gain and provide optimum return on resources invested (Department of Health, 1997b).

THE EMERGENCE OF QUALITY OF LIFE
AS AN OUTCOME MEASURE IN HEALTH CARE

Before 1970, health care researchers were, by and large, content to focus either on major morbidity and mortality or on measures of physiological function or patient functional performance as indicators of health gain. Improvements in cardiac, pulmonary or renal function, metabolic indices or laboratory exercise capacity were used to justify therapeutic interventions. However, the ultimate aims of treating patients are to make them live longer and/or better. During the past 20 or 30 years, there has been an increasing realisation that surrogate indices such as the physiological parameters outlined above are inadequate when used to determine whether patients' lives are improved by therapy (Guyatt and Cook, 1994; Joyce, O'Boyle and McGee, 1998). In addition to their biological effects, illnesses, diseases and their treatments can have a significant impact on such areas of function as mobility, mood, life satisfaction, sexuality, cognition, and ability to fulfil occupational, social and family roles. Health status measurement has evolved to allow insight into patients' experiences in these areas and quality of life has emerged as a broad term to describe this domain of measurement. The quality of life construct may be viewed as a paradigm shift in the measurement of health gain, since it shifts the focus of attention from symptoms to functioning and establishes the primacy, or at least the legitimacy, of the patient perspective (Leplege and Hunt, 1997).

USES OF QUALITY OF LIFE DATA

Among the most important and basic questions about quality of life in health care are: Why should it be studied and what data support its use? These questions may be addressed from the perspective of a patient, carer, nurse, physician, drug company, health board or even a country. The answer is most obvious for the individual patient: quality of life studies can help improve the quality of care. High quality care may be defined as:

> care that is desired by informed patients (and family); is based on sound judgement of the professionals involved from scientific studies and/or experience; and is agreed upon and carried out in a relationship of mutual understanding and respect (Williams, 1996).

Quality of life data are relevant in relation to all three components of this definition. For example, in providing information to patients, quality of life data may be used to differentiate between two therapies that show marginal differences in their impact on mortality or morbidity. Quality of life data may have important impacts on prescribing practices and this is reflected in the growing interest in such studies within the pharmaceutical industry (Spilker, 1996). Quality of life assessment is particularly relevant to patients with progressive conditions, especially in the later phases of disease (O'Boyle, 1996; O'Boyle and Waldron, 1997). For a health board or a country's health planners, the most important use of quality of life data is to improve resource allocation.

WHAT IS QUALITY OF LIFE?

There is enormous current interest in the developed and developing world in quality of life (Bowling, 1995; Spilker, 1996; Walker and Rosser, 1993). However, quality of life is an amorphous construct that has a usage across many disciplines. There are a variety of definitions, including crude attempts at quantification. Because quality of life is such a vague concept, with such a multitude of usages, the definition is often more dependent on the user and in particular their understanding and agenda (Leplege and Hunt, 1997; Joyce, O'Boyle and McGee, 1998). A good example of this is the Irish Department of Health's Cancer Strategy Document (1996) which lists the aim:

> to ensure that those who develop cancer receive the most effective care and treatment and that their quality of life is enhanced to the greatest possible extent.

This early reference to enhanced quality of life is not further developed in the document except in relation to palliative care and could be seen as representing something of a pious aspiration in which the term quality of life is used more as a cliché rather than a scientific construct amenable to measurement and explication. A critical appraisal of quality of life measurements (Gill and Feinstein, 1994) highlights the problem of conceptualisation and definition. Investigators defined what they meant by the term quality of life in only 11 (15 per cent) of the 75 articles reviewed; identified the targeted domains in only 35 (47 per cent); and gave reasons for selecting the chosen quality of life instruments in only 27 (36 per cent). No investigator distinguished "overall" quality of life from health-related quality of life. The measures used focused on predefined areas rather than allowing patients to define the areas that they themselves considered to be important. Patients were invited to give their own specific rating of quality of life in only 13 studies (17 per cent), were asked to supplement the stipulated items with personal responses in only nine (13 per cent) and to rate the importance of individual items in only six (8.5 per cent).

REFINING THE CONCEPT OF QUALITY OF LIFE

Two perspectives assist in refining the concept of quality of life: health outcomes and health-related quality of life.

Health Outcomes

In health care, quality of life is best understood, although not exclusively, in the context of health outcomes. The usually cited definition of a health outcome is "a change in a patient's current and future health status that can be attributed to antecedent health care" (Donabedian, 1985). Outcome indicators have traditionally included such measures as avoidable mortality, standardised mortality ratios, hospital re-admission and other service use indicators, laboratory investigations, diagnostic tests, morbidity, case severity, adverse reactions, complications, technical success, symptom relief, pain and cost-effectiveness. All of these are, of course, important and provide relevant information. They do, however, implicitly represent a biomedical model of disease that is increasingly being seen as inadequate since it provides little scope for input by the patient.

The biomedical model is rooted in a belief that ill health is an objective, measurable state. This is a disease-based view of ill health in which poor health is a function of an abnormality. Illness is a different concept. It refers to a person's subjective experience of ill health and is indicated by reported symptoms and subjective accounts in terms of pain, distress and discomfort. The doctor and the patient come to the medical process with different models, the disease model and the illness model, which must be integrated if the outcome is to be successful. One way to achieve this is to incorporate patient-generated assessments such as quality of life measures into the clinical process.

Although some investigators are sceptical about patient-based in-dicators of outcome, there are a number of important arguments for including such measures. First, the goals of the medical and health sciences are to add years to life *and* life to years. When the condition is incurable, the goal is to ensure the best possible quality of life for the patient. There are many examples of studies which have reported low levels of agreement among doctors and between doctors' and patients' judgements (Spangers and Aaronson, 1992). Incorporating patient-based outcomes refocuses efforts on a more holistic set of treatment goals and provides a patient-centred baseline for assess-ment of treatment.

Health-related Quality of Life

The second approach to refining the concept of quality of life is to restrict its definition to health-related quality of life. Because of the amorphous and multidimensional nature of quality of life, most re-searchers in medicine and health care concern themselves with a sub-component of quality of life, which has been termed health-related quality of life. This is distinguished from quality of life as a whole, which would also include such components as adequacy of educa-tion, housing, income and perceptions of the immediate environ-ment. Patrick and Erickson (1993) define health-related quality of life as:

> the value assigned to the duration of life as modified by the social opportunities, perceptions, functional states and im-pairments that are influenced by disease, injuries, treatments or policy.

There is broad agreement that, in measuring health-related quality of life, we should assess a number of crucial areas, including physical function, psychological state, somatic symptoms such as pain, social function including relationships, sexual function and occupational function and possibly financial state. We should include some as-sessment of the patient's level of general wellbeing and of satisfac-tion with treatment, outcome and health status and with future pros-pects.

The concept of health-related quality of life owes much to the original World Health Organisation (WHO) definition of health as a state of complete physical, mental and social wellbeing and not merely the absence of disease (WHO, 1948). The WHO established a working party which is undertaking a ten-country study of quality of life. The WHOQoL group has provided the following definition of quality of life:

> Quality of life is defined as the individual's perception of their position in life in the context of the culture and value systems in which they live and in relation to their goals, expectations, standards and concerns. It is a broad ranging concept affected in a complex way by a person's physical health, psychological state, level of independence and their relationships to salient features of their environment (Szabo, 1996).

This definition underpins the development of the WHOQoL as a core measure, specific editions of which are planned for various groups such as cancer patients (Szabo, 1996).

The restriction of quality of life assessment to health-related quality of life and the use of health status measures to assess this is not entirely satisfactory. Most questionnaires now referred to as health-related quality of life measures are really former measures of health status in a new guise and place an overwhelming reliance on the assessment of functional capacity. As such, while purporting to incorporate the patients' perspectives, they implicitly represent the medical model, which stresses the ability to perform everyday tasks and fulfil social and occupational roles. Such measures ignore the meaning and importance of such tasks and roles for the individual and, under the guise of obtaining the patients' perceptions, act to preserve the supremacy of professional judgements, leading to the suppression of what is supposed to be under scrutiny (Joyce, 1988; Leplege and Hunt, 1997).

FUTURE DIRECTIONS IN QUALITY OF LIFE RESEARCH

The next section of this chapter focuses on a number of themes that are likely to become increasingly important in quality of life research.

First, the questions of how quality of life should be assessed, and in particular the need for individualised assessment, are briefly addressed. Second, the importance of carers and the need to reconcile different perspectives are highlighted. Third, the impact of ageing of the population for quality of life research is addressed and the particular importance of quality of life assessment in palliative care is discussed. Finally, a brief discussion of the likely future importance of quality of life measures in formulating health policy is presented.

How Should Quality of Life Be Measured?

The concepts underlying quality of life are complex and multidimensional and this has resulted in both differing conceptualisations and a wide variety of measurement techniques, which reflect the lack of agreement on definition. In general, measurement of quality of life in medicine and health care is guided by two principles: multidimensionality and subjectivity. Most authors recommend that a comprehensive evaluation should cover several key domains: physical symptoms, physical role and social functioning, psychological distress, cognitive function, body image and sexual functioning (Bowling, 1991; 1995). These are usually assessed by asking the patient to complete subjective questionnaires, or by a health care professional or relative making a proxy assessment.

In choosing a measure, or set of measures, the key questions are whether a disease-specific measure or a generic measure is needed and whether either requires supplementation with single-domain measures that are important to the study aims. Examples of generic measures are the well-known Sickness Impact Profile, The Nottingham Health Questionnaire, the McMaster Health Index and the SF-36, which are now very widely used. The Nottingham Health Questionnaire, for example, provides the patient with the opportunity to rate symptoms such as fatigue, pain, anxiety and depression and also the extent to which their health is causing problems in work, social life, sex life and so on. Such measures can provide important information about the impact of medical and surgical interventions. One problem with general measures such as these is that they may not be specific enough to capture small but significant changes in health status or levels of disease severity. This has led to the development of a host of disease-specific quality of life measures (Bowling, 1995). A combined approach, in which a generic measure such as the SF-36 is used together with a disease-specific measure, is increasingly the norm.

The Need for an Individual Perspective

Questionnaire approaches to the measurement of quality of life provide important information. However, such measures impose a predetermined value system on the respondent. Someone other than the respondent has decided which questions to ask, which areas should be explored and which areas should not be addressed. Furthermore, the relative importance assigned to the patient's answers, as reflected in the weightings which must be applied to obtain a score, may not, indeed are likely not to be those which the patient would use (Cohen, 1982; Joyce et al., 1998). In assessing quality of life, it is particularly important to know at any given time what particular issues are of most concern to the patient (Hayry, 1991). We have previously proposed a phenomenological approach to quality of life — that is, one which focuses on the individual's personal view of life and of its quality (Joyce, 1988; O'Boyle, 1992; 1994; O'Boyle et al., 1992; 1993). We have suggested that quality of life should be defined as what the individual determines it to be. Similarly, Hayry (1991) has proposed that "the quality, or value, of an individual's life is no more and no less than what she considers it to be".

Calman (1984) proposed an important model for the assessment of quality of life which again places the emphasis on the perspective of the individual. Quality of life is the difference, at a particular period in time, between the hopes and expectations of the individual and their present experience. It depends on the individual's past experience, present lifestyle and personal hopes and ambitions for the future. The gap between hopes and realities may be narrowed by improving the patient's functions (reality) through treatment or by reducing expectations through informed understanding of the limitations of their disease and acceptance of the risks involved in treatment in relation to expected benefits.

One way of addressing the individual nature of quality of life is to use measures designed to assess quality of life from the unique perspective of the individual. One such measure is the Schedule for the Evaluation of Individual Quality of Life (O'Boyle et al., 1993). The SEIQoL, which was developed in Ireland, is now in use in over 200 centres worldwide. It measures three elements of quality of life: what areas of life are important to the respondent; how they are currently doing in each of these areas; and what is the relative importance of each of these areas to them. This approach has been successfully used in a number of applications in Ireland, including hip replacement surgery, HIV/AIDS treatment, care of the elderly and, as discussed below, palliative care (O'Boyle, 1994; 1997; O'Boyle et al., 1992; 1993; 1995). Quality of life scores generated by the measures, for a number of patient populations studied in Ireland, are shown in Table 8.1. Other measures have been designed which seek to incorporate the unique perspective of the individual patient (Joyce et al., 1998). These include the Patient Generated Index (Ruta et al., 1994), the Repertory Grid Technique (Thunedborg et al., 1993; Dunbar et al., 1992) and the Quality of Life Index (Ferrans and Powers, 1985).

Table 8.1: SEIQoL Mean Global Scores (Standard Deviation) for a Number of Irish Patient Populations

Population	Mean SEIQoL Score	Standard Deviation	Mean SEIQoL Score	Standard Deviation
Healthy elderly	82.1	(12.2)		
Healthy young	77.4	(9.5)		
Peptic Ulcer Disease	72.6	(12.6)		
Irritable Bowel Syndrome	62.9	(17.4)		
Elderly Arthritis	61.6	(18.8)	70.7*	(11.2)*
Elderly Arthritis	60.7	(9.4)	58.9**	(5.6)**
Palliative care	60.4	(17.5)		

* These patients were reassessed 7.5 months after hip replacement surgery.
** These control arthritis patients were also reassessed after 7.5 months.

Source: O'Boyle et al. (1993).

Differing Perspectives

It is important to understand the limitations of health care professionals in accurately judging patient's concerns (Presant, 1984). Spangers and Aaronson (1992), in a review of the literature on proxy ratings of quality of life, concluded that agreement between patients' self-ratings and those of health care providers and of relatives was generally poor. Early so-called quality of life measures, such as the Karnofsky Scale and the Spitzer Scales, were rated solely by the doctor (Karnofsky et al., 1949; Spitzer et al., 1981). Slevin et al. (1988) showed that agreement between doctors' and patients' ratings on these scales was poor. With the emergence of data such as these showing discrepancies between doctors', nurses' and patient ratings, the importance of patient ratings increased. Agreement between ratings depends on a number of factors: level of concreteness and visibility of the domain rated; type of rater; relationship to patient; closeness of living arrangement with patient. One of the major challenges facing this type of outcomes research is how to aggregate the various types of outcome measure. There is broad agreement that traditional outcome measures such as signs and symptoms must be complemented with patient-centred measures such as health status and quality of life. As shown in Table 8.2, the emphasis may vary depending on the context in which the measures are applied.

Quality of Life and Ageing

The world's population is ageing. In 1900, there were 10–17 million people aged 65 or older, constituting less than one per cent of the total population. By 1992, there were 342 million people in the over-65 age group, making up 6.2 per cent of the population. By the year 2050, the number of people aged 65 or older will expand to at least 2.5 billion — about a fifth of the world's projected population (Olshansky et al., 1993). Ireland will not be immune to these changes. According to the 1996 Census (Central Statistics Office, 1997) there were 413,882 persons aged 65 years and over living in the Republic of Ireland, representing 11.4 per cent of the general population. While the overall State population is expected to remain stable, the number

Table 8.2: Levels of Disease and Treatment Outcome in Cancer*

Level of Outcome	Example of Measure	Disease Progression	Curative Treatment	Palliative Treatment
Pathological process/signs	Tumour volume CAT/MRI scan	Increase	Decrease	Little impact
Symptoms	McGill pain scale	Likely increase	Decrease	Decrease
Side-effects	Self-report scale	–	Aim to minimise	Aim to minimise
Health status: specific	EORTC Scales	Likely decrease	Aim to increase	Aim to increase
Health status: generic	SF36	Likely decrease	Aim to increase	Aim to increase
Quality of life	SEIQoL	Likely decrease, but with adaptation could stay constant or even increase	Aim to achieve pre-level	Aim to maximise
Cost	Various criteria, e.g. Treatment cost, QALY cost			

* The relative importance of the different levels of outcome will vary with the particular condition, patient and approach to management. Palliative treatment, for example, may have little impact on the pathological process, would aim to decrease symptoms with minimal side-effects, while increasing health status (function) and maximising quality of life at an acceptable economic cost.

of elderly will grow by almost 107,771 in the period 1996 to 2011, and will represent 14.1 per cent of the general population by the year 2011 (Fahey, 1995). A high proportion of this increase will occur in populations with traditionally high levels of need for health and social care services. Almost 33,000 more people aged 70 or older are expected to be living alone in the year 2011 compared to 1991, representing a 47 per cent increase in the over-70s population living alone. The number of people aged 80 years or more is expected to increase by 51,000 over this period. This represents a two-thirds increase in both elderly men and women aged 80 and over in this period.

Quality of life outcomes will assume increasing importance in health for a number of reasons associated with the ageing of the population (O'Boyle, 1997). Three epidemiological scenarios may result from the demographic change which is likely to occur (Fries, 1992). First, the average period of morbidity experienced before death may increase if medical interventions do not affect the onset of chronic disease but only delay mortality (the "failure of success" scenario). Second, the average age of onset of chronic disease as well as mortality may increase, resulting in no change in the average period of morbidity. Third, the average age of onset for chronic disease may be postponed due to changes in lifestyle, with no change or a slow increase in longevity (the compression of morbidity hypothesis). There is considerable debate about which of these scenarios is most likely to occur but all have significant consequences for health care. The compression of morbidity hypothesis suggests that an increasing proportion of elderly people will spend an increasing proportion of their old age in good health with good quality of life. Social and health care policies for this population will then need to be aimed at maintaining or enhancing quality of life. There is renewed interest worldwide in what may be termed "successful ageing". It has been proposed that efforts to meet the needs of elderly people should focus on three factors: their economic security, their psychosocial well-being and their perceived health (O'Boyle, 1997).

The compression of morbidity hypothesis has been challenged by many scientists who posit an expansion of morbidity (Olshansky et al., 1993). It is argued that behavioural factors such as diet and exercise, which are known to reduce the risk of fatal illnesses, do not change the onset or progression of most debilitating diseases associated with ageing. We have already seen significant increases in chronic conditions such as heart disease, hypertension, various forms of cancer, stroke, diabetes and arthritis and this trend is likely to continue with the ageing of the population. Some data indicate that the average number of years that people spend disabled has grown faster than the average number of years they spend healthy (Olshansky et al., 1993). As new medical technologies are developed which seek to postpone death, increasing numbers of people will live longer periods in states of disability. If this happens, a shift in resources will be required to ensure that services will be available to maximise the quality of life of such people. This would require a major refocusing of health care, which is largely oriented at present towards expensive acute care interventions, to the provision of long-term care, the need for which will rapidly increase as the population ages. Ethically difficult issues will emerge relating to end-of-life care (Lancet, 1992). How widely will technologies to maintain life at all costs be used and what limits and criteria will be applied? In such scenarios, the availability of empirically based quality of life data will prove essential (O'Boyle, 1996; 1997; O'Boyle and Waldron, 1997).

Older people are relatively heavy users of health services. In Ireland, those aged over 65 have nearly twice as many GP visits per year as the overall population, with usage being particularly high in those over 75 (Nolan, 1991). However, Fahey (1995; see also Chapter 11 in this volume) concluded that the growth in the number of older people has a weaker and more uncertain influence on the demand for health services than might be expected. The demographic effect is smaller than that which derives from economic growth and the consequent increase in purchasing power in the economy. It is also less important than a wide range of institutional influences on the health services such as government policy and attempts to control government health spending and the actions of dominant interest groups such as medical professionals, health insurers and drug companies. Rather than look at demographic trends as a determinant of health service requirements, Fahey proposes that it might be more useful for policy-making to refer to demographic indicators as a measure of effectiveness of health policy. While demographic measures, particularly those related to life expectancy and mortality, have much to offer as indicators of health gain in this context, so also do measures of health status and quality of life.

Quality of Life in Palliative Care

Most authors who have considered palliative care have placed quality of life centre-stage as the primary outcome to be assessed. The Department of Health, in the National Cancer Strategy, accepts that palliative care is concerned primarily with quality of life, but provides no rationale either for measuring or maximising quality of life in palliative care settings. The old management adage that "if you can't measure it, you can't manage it" would seem to apply. In this context, it is noteworthy that a key goal of the Department is to assist in the development of an enhanced capacity within the health system to deal with emerging medico-legal and ethical issues (Department of Health, 1994). There is an urgent need to develop and implement acceptable measures of quality of life in palliative care, not only to assess outcome but also to assist in the increasingly complex ethical dilemmas which are arising in this type of medical setting, where end-of-life decisions are often based on a judgement about quality of life.

There are some special considerations that apply to the assessment of quality of life in palliative care (O'Boyle and Waldron, 1997). Valid and reliable scientific data may be difficult to collect, particularly in the later stages of care. Families are intimately involved in palliative care and provide both a source of information and an important focus of treatment which is aimed at maintaining not only the best quality of life for the patient but also for the family. The intricate relationships between physical and psychological factors in terminal illness are significantly under-researched and the mechanisms of human adaptation in progressive disease are little understood. Finally, issues such as end-of-life decisions create complex medico-legal and ethical webs in which society expects guidance not only from the judiciary but also from the medical and nursing professions. Such decisions are usually (invariably?) based on quality of life concerns.

Individually based quality of life measures are particularly suitable for palliative care. We have recently reported preliminary findings from the first study applying the SEIQoL in palliative care (Waldron et al., 1995). An important finding was the very high validity and reliability outcomes which indicated that patients receiving palliative care have a particularly deep insight into their quality of life. While the SEIQoL was found to be acceptable in the palliative care setting, is likely to be too complex for routine use. A simpler direct method of determining the relative importance of the different areas of life nominated by patients (Hickey et al., 1996; Browne et al., 1997) is currently under investigation in palliative care.

Quality of life has heretofore been considered solely as an outcome measure. However, developments in psychoneuroimmunology and evidence from a number of clinical studies raise the intriguing possibility that quality of life might influence pathological processes such as tumour progression (Coates et al., 1987; Ganz et al., 1991; Maltori et al., 1995; Spiegel et al., 1989). If this were to be the case, then interventions aimed at maximising patient quality of life might also influence disease progression.

QUALITY OF LIFE AND HEALTH POLICY

Health decision-making has never been more important, whether to reduce inefficiency, eliminate ineffective medical procedures, increase competition, improve quality, change reimbursement formulas or ration limited resources and services. Assessment of quality of life and health status is playing an increasing role in the development and implementation of health policy in a number of countries, and this trend is likely to increase (Williams, 1996). Increasingly, decision-makers, providers, patients and the public ask that every additional expenditure be justified according to expected outcomes.

In addressing the costs and benefits of services, the use of measures of health status and health-related quality of life are increasingly being advocated (Patrick and Erickson, 1993, 1996). The Unites States Congress established the Agency for Health Care Policy and Research to undertake research on the effectiveness of medical care in terms of its impact on patient outcomes, including quality of life and health status. The FDA encourages the collection of quality of life data for new drugs. In the UK, quality of life, health status and the experiences of patients and carers are explicitly included in outcome assessment (Department of Health (UK), 1992).

The Irish Department of Health, in its strategy document *Shaping a Healthier Future* (1994), proposed that:

> The concepts of health gain and social gain, allied to greatly improved data collection and analysis, will be used to focus

the prevention, treatment and care more clearly on improvements in health status or quality of life.

Both health gain and social gain underline the need for a demonstrable benefit from the health services, while recognising that the benefit in question may be difficult to measure. These developments suggest a new vision of the future in which the value of health care services is measured from the patient's perspective in terms of how services make a difference in people's day-to-day living, complementing traditional measures such as disease state and mortality.

The difficulties associated with obtaining valid and reliable measures of health status and quality of life and of incorporating these into decision-making should not be underestimated. The importance of doing this cannot be overestimated. In discussing the proposed approach to these problems, the Department of Health:

> promises that decisions on priorities and the allocation of resources will be made in a more open and objective way and will draw in particular on detailed information and analysis of needs, costs and outcomes. However, the priority setting process can never be entirely objective. One can establish the potential benefits to be derived from different types of services, but a subjective decision still needs to be made in relation to the relative value of these benefits. It may be possible to measure, for example, the health gain from cardiac surgery and from joint replacements; it may be possible to measure the social gain deriving from better support services for the parents of children with mental handicap living in the community. But how are these quite different benefits to be ranked in determining where extra resources are to be made available? There is a tendency for such choices to be made in an arbitrary way and mainly in the interests of those groups able to exert the most influence over the resource allocation process. This is very much in conflict with the principle of equity. . . . Identifying public preferences between competing priorities is crucial to opening up the process and making the choice mechanisms more explicit (Department of Health, 1994).

Incorporating the Consumer's Perspective

Incorporating public preferences into decisions about priority setting will require, in addition to traditional measures of outcome, detailed assessments of health status and quality of life across a broad range of conditions. Integrating the various levels of outcome will pose a significant challenge for health services research. Table 8.2 shows an attempt to integrate the more traditional outcomes such as signs and symptoms with the more modern outcomes such as health status and quality of life for curative and palliative care at the level of the individual patient. Clearly, the complexity increases as one moves from the individual patient to the group or population level and some rationale will be needed to determine the emphasis to be placed on the various outcomes in prioritising health care.

Given sufficient acceptance of the importance of the consumer's perspective in health care delivery, quality of life studies could contribute to health policy in a number of ways by providing, for example:

- Policy-relevant information for the purposes of medical and surgical audit;

- Information to inform consumers regarding treatment choices and their likely outcomes;

- Information relevant to the design of insurance policies, design of benefits, organisation of health care providers and reform of payment systems.

Policy decisions need to be based upon sound empirical data. Data from oncology studies show that there can be significant differences of opinion between providers and recipients of care. For example, Slevin et al. (1990) found that patients with cancer were much more likely to opt for radical treatment with minimal chance of benefit than people who do not have cancer, including medical and nursing professionals. Coates et al. (1987) found, unexpectedly, that continuous chemotherapy was superior to intermittent chemotherapy in improving the quality of life of patients. Earl et al. (1991) studied a group of patients with small cell carcinoma of the lung and random-

ised them to receive either regular "planned" chemotherapy or chemotherapy given "as required". Contrary to expectations, the "as required" patient group scored themselves as having more severe
symptoms than patients receiving planned treatment. Sugarbaker et
al. (1982) found that their hypothesis that limb-sparing surgery plus
irradiation would provide improved quality of life in patients with
limb sarcoma, when compared to amputation, was not sustained.
These studies highlight the need for supplementing the judgements
of health professionals with properly generated patient-centred data.

Quality of life studies complement the increasing emphasis on
patient autonomy and informed consent. Competent and autonomous patients need to and will make decisions, including end-of-life
decisions, based, *inter alia*, on their evaluation of the implications for
their quality of life. Ideological struggles can occur between providers who adopt a rational objective approach to quality of life, and
patients who view quality of life in terms of their unique personal
situation. Considerable suffering in one domain may be overridden
by an enhanced sense of personal meaning in another resulting in a
net increase in quality of life despite coexisting suffering. On the
other hand, the Anti-D debacle has shown the enormous cost in
terms of suffering and impairment in quality of life that can occur
when things go wrong in a health care service.

Consideration of patient quality of life promotes improved clinical
interventions, assists in treatment comparisons and will prove increasingly important in the identification of services and facilities
and in resource allocation. The various methodologies derived to
measure quality of life offer the potential for a final common path-
way for assessing the multidisciplinary inputs of basic scientists and
clinicians to diagnostic and treatment processes. As such, quality of
life could become the dominant criterion by which health care decisions are made and health gain is judged. We should not, however,
underestimate the challenges that must be faced and the difficulties
that must be overcome to incorporate such patient-centred measures
into decision-making at all levels of health care. We need to assess
quality of life because it places the patient at the heart of the thera-

peutic process. Having reviewed the literature on quality of life, Gill and Feinstein (1994) concluded

> that quality of life is a uniquely personal perception, denoting the way that individuals feel about their health status and/or non-medical aspects of their lives. . . . most measurements of quality of life seem to aim at the wrong target. . . . quality of life can be suitably measured only by determining the opinions of patients and by supplementing (or replacing) the instruments developed by "experts".

References

Bowling, A. (1991), *Measuring Health: A Review of Quality of Life Measurement Scales*, Milton Keynes: Open University Press.

Bowling, A. (1995), *Measuring Disease: A Review of Disease-Specific Quality of Life Measurement Scales*, Milton Keynes: Open University Press.

Browne, J.P., C.A. O'Boyle, H.M. McGee, N.J. McDonald, and C.R.B. Joyce (1997), "Development of a Direct Weighting Procedure for Quality of Life Domains", *Quality of Life Research*, Vol. 6, pp. 301–9.

Calman, K.C. (1984), "Quality of Life in Cancer Patients — an Hypothesis", *Journal of Medical Ethics*, Vol. 10, pp. 124–7.

Central Statistics Office (1997), *Census 96: Principal Demographic Results*, Dublin: Stationery Office.

Coates, A., V. Gebski, J.F. Bishop, P.N. Jeal et al. (1987), "Improving the Quality of Life during Chemotherapy for Advanced Breast Cancer", *New England Journal of Medicine*, Vol. 317, pp. 1490–5.

Cohen, C. (1982), "On the Quality of Life: some Philosophical Reflections", *Circulation*, Vol. 66 (Supplement 3), pp. 29–33.

Department of Health (Irl) (1994), *Shaping a Healthier Future*, Dublin: Government Publications Office.

Department of Health (Irl) (1996), *Cancer Services in Ireland: A National Strategy* Dublin: Government Publications Office.

Department of Health (Irl) (1997), *Statement on Strategy* Dublin: Government Publications Office.

Department of Health (Irl) (1997), *A Plan for Women's Health for the Years 1997–1999*, Dublin: Government Publications Office.

Department of Health (UK) (1992), *Assessing the Effects of Health Technologies: Principles, Practice and Proposals*, London: HMSO.

Donabedian, A. (1985), *Explorations in Quality Assessment and Monitoring*, Vols. 1–3, Ann Arbor, MI: Health Administration Press.

Dunbar, G.C., M.J. Stoker, T.C.P. Hodges, and G. Beaumont (1992), "The Development of SBQoL — a Unique Scale for Measuring Quality of Life", *British Journal of Medical Economics*, Vol. 2, pp. 65–74.

Earl, H.M., R.M. Rudd, S.G. Spiro, C.M. Ash, L.E. James, C.S. Law et al. (1991), "A Randomised Trial of Planned versus As Required Chemotherapy in Small Cell Lung Cancer: a Cancer Research Campaign Trial", *British Journal of Cancer*, Vol. 64, pp. 566–72.

Fahey, T. (1995), "Health and Social Care Implications of Population Ageing in Ireland 1991–2001", Report No. 42, Dublin: National Council for the Elderly.

Ferrans, C.E. and M.J. Powers (1985), "Quality of Life Index: Development and Psychometric Properties", *American Journal of Nursing Science*, Vol. 8, pp. 15–24.

Fries, J.F. (1992), "Strategies for Reduction of Morbidity", *American Journal of Clinical Nutrition*, Vol. 55, pp. 1257–62.

Ganz, P.A., J. Lee and J. Siau (1991), "Quality of Life Assessment: an Independent Prognostic Variable for Survival in Lung Cancer", *Cancer*, Vol. 67, pp. 3131–5.

Gill, T.M. and A.R. Feinstein (1994), "A Critical Appraisal of the Quality of Quality-of-Life Measurements", *Journal of American Medical Association*, Vol. 272, pp. 619–26.

Guyatt, G.H. and D.J. Cook (1994), "Health Status, Quality of Life and the Individual", *Journal of the American Medical Association*, Vol. 272, pp. 630–1.

Hayry, M. (1991), "Measuring the Quality of Life: Why, How and What?", *Theoretical Medicine*, Vol. 12, pp. 97–116.

Hickey, A., G. Bury, C.A. O'Boyle, F. Bradley, F.D. O'Kelly and W. Shannon (1996), "A New Short Form Quality of Life Measure (SEIQoL-DW): Application in a Cohort of Individuals with HIV/AIDS", *British Medical Journal*, Vol. 313, pp. 29–33.

Joyce, C.R.B. (1988), "Quality of Life: the State of the Art in Clinical Assessment" in S.R. Walker and R.M. Rosser (eds.), *Quality of Life: Assessment and Application*, Lancaster: MTP Press.

Joyce, C.R.B., C.A. O'Boyle and H.M. McGee (eds.) (1998), *Individual Quality of Life: Approaches to Conceptualisation and Measurement in Health*, London: Harwood Academic Press (in press).

Karnofsky, D.A. and J.H. Burchenal (1949), "The Clinical Evaluation of Chemotherapeutic Agents in Cancer" in C.M. McLeod (ed.), *Evaluation of Chemotherapeutic Agents*, New York: Columbia University Press.

Lancet, The (1992), "Advance Directives", *The Lancet*, Vol. 340, pp. 1321–2.

Leplege, A. and S. Hunt (1997), "The Problem of Quality of Life", *Journal of the American Medical Association*, Vol. 278, pp. 47–50.

Maltori, M., M. Pirovano, E. Scrapi, M. Marinari, M. Indelli, M.D. Arnoldi et al. (1995), "Prediction of Survival of Patients Terminally Ill with Cancer", *Cancer*, Vol. 75, pp. 2613–22.

Nolan, B. (1991), "Utilisation and Financing of the Health Services in Ireland" Dublin: Economic and Social Research Institute.

O'Boyle, C.A. (1992), "Assessment of Quality of Life in Surgery", *British Journal of Surgery*, Vol. 79, pp. 395–8.

O'Boyle, C.A. (1994), "The Schedule for the Evaluation of Individual Quality of Life", *International Journal of Mental Health*, Vol. 23, No. 3, pp. 3–23.

O'Boyle, C.A. (1996), "Quality of Life in Palliative Care" in G. Ford and I. Lewin (eds.), *Managing Terminal Illness*, London: RCP Publications, pp. 37–47.

O'Boyle, C.A. (1997), "Measuring the Quality of Later Life", *Philosophical Transactions of the Royal Society, London*, Vol. 352, pp. 1871–9.

O'Boyle, C.A., H.M. McGee, A. Hickey, C.R.B. Joyce et al. (1993), *The Schedule for the Evaluation of Individual Quality of Life: User Manual*, Dublin: Department of Psychology, Royal College of Surgeons in Ireland.

O'Boyle, C. A., H.M. McGee, A. Hickey, K. O'Malley and C.R.B. Joyce (1992), "Individual Quality of Life in Patients Undergoing Hip Replacement", *Lancet*, Vol. 339, pp. 1088–91.

O'Boyle, C.A., H. McGee and C.R.B. Joyce (1995), "Quality of Life: Assessing the Individual" in G.L. Albrecht and R. Fitzpatrick (eds.), *Quality of Life in Health Care: Advances in Medical Sociology*, Vol. 5, Greenwich, CT: JAI Press, pp. 159–80.

O'Boyle, C.A. and D. Waldron (1997), "Quality of Life Issues in Palliative Medicine", *Journal of Neurology*, Vol. 244, pp. S18–25.

Olshansky, S.J., B.A. Carnes and C.K. Cassel (1993), "The Ageing of the Human Species", *Scientific American*, Vol. 268, pp. 18–24.

Patrick, D.L. and P. Erickson (1993), "Assessing Health-related Quality of Life for Clinical Decision-making" in S.R. Walker and R.M. Rosser (eds.), *Quality of Life Assessment: Key Issues for the 1990s*, London: Kluwer Academic Press, pp.11–64.

Patrick, D.L. and P. Erickson (1996), "Applications of Health Status Assessment to Health Policy" in B. Spilker (ed.), *Quality of Life and Pharmacoeconomics in Clinical Trials*, Second Edition, Philadelphia, PA: Lippincott-Raven Publishers, pp. 717–27.

Presant, C.A. (1984), "Quality of Life in Cancer Patients: Who Measures What?" *American Journal of Clinical Oncology* (CCT), Vol. 7, pp. 571–3.

Ruta, D.A., A.M. Garratt, M. Leng, I.T. Russell and L.M. McDonald (1994), "A New Approach to the Measurement of Quality of Life: the Patient Generated Index", *Medical Care*, Vol. 32, pp. 1109–26.

Slevin, M.L., H. Plant, D. Lynch, J. Drinkwater and W.M. Gregory (1988), "Who Should Measure Quality of Life, the Doctor or the Patient?" *British Journal of Cancer*, Vol. 57, pp. 109–12.

Slevin, M.L, L. Stubbs, H.J. Plant, P. Wilson et al. (1990), "Attitudes to Chemotherapy: Comparing Views of Patients with Cancer with those of Doctors, Nurses and General Practitioners", *British Medical Journal*, Vol. 300, pp. 1458–60.

Spangers, M.A.G. and N.K. Aaronson (1992), "The Role of Health Care Providers and Significant Others in Evaluating the Quality of Life of Patients with Chronic Disease: a Review", *Clinical Epidemiology*, Vol. 45, pp. 743–60.

Spiegel, D., J.R. Bloom, H.C. Kramer and E. Gottheil (1989), "Effect of Psychosocial Treatment on Survival of Patients with Metastatic Breast Cancer", *Lancet*, Vol. 14, 888–91.

Spilker, B. (ed.) (1990), "Quality of Life Assessments" in *Clinical Trials*, New York: Raven Press.

Spilker, B. (ed.) (1996), *Quality of Life and Pharmacoeconomics in Clinical Trials*, Second Edition, Philadelphia, PA: Lippincott-Raven Publishers.

Spitzer, W.O., A.J. Dobson, J. Hall, E. Chesterman et al. (1981), "Measuring the Quality of Life of Cancer Patients: a Concise ql-index for Use by Physicians", *Journal of Chronic Diseases*, Vol. 34, pp. 585–97.

Sugarbaker, P.H., I. Barofsky, S.A. Rosenberg and F.J. Gianola (1982), "Quality of Life Assessment of Patients in Extremity Sarcoma Clinical Trials", *Surgery*, Vol. 91, pp. 17–23.

Szabo, S. (1996), "The World Health Organisation Quality of Life Assessment Instrument" in B. Spilker (ed.), *Quality of Life and Pharmacoeconomics in Clinical Trials*, Second Edition, Philadelphia, PA: Lippincott-Raven Publishers, pp. 355–62.

Thunedborg, K., P. Allerup, P. Bech and C.R.B. Joyce (1993), "Development of the Repertory Grid for Measurement of Individual Quality of Life in Clinical Trials", *International Journal of Methods in Psychiatric Research*, Vol. 3, pp. 45–56.

Waldron, D., C.A. O'Boyle, M. Moriarty, M. Kearney, and D. Carney (1995), "Use of an Individualised Measure of Quality of Life, the SEIQoL, in Palliative Care: Results of a Pilot Study", Paper presented to the Annual Meeting of the Palliative Care Research Forum, Durham, 8 November.

Walker, S.R. and R.M. Rosser (1993), *Quality of Life Assessment: Key Issues for the 1990s*, London: Kluwer Academic Press.

Williams, A.H. (1996), "Health Policy Implications of Using Quality of Life Measures in the Economic Evaluation of Health Care" in B. Spilker (ed.), *Quality of Life and Pharmacoeconomics in Clinical Trials*, Second Edition, Philadelphia, PA: Lippincott-Raven Publishers, pp. 753–60.

World Health Organisation (1948), *Constitution of the World Health Organisation: Basic Documents*, Geneva: World Health Organisation.

9

DEVELOPMENT AND ASSESSMENT OF MEDICAL TECHNOLOGY

Yunnus Gul and *Ara Darzi*

INTRODUCTION

The field of medicine is changing fundamentally and this has been made possible by advances in medical technology and industrial achievement. Developmental trends in such technology indicate that we are entering an exciting era of advanced medical care, as heralded by the development and progress in minimal access surgery, which has been regarded as one of the great innovations of health care in the 1990s. In the next century, technology will not only change processes but, on another level, will alter the structure of the health service. This chapter opens with a discussion of examples of developments that will alter surgical processes. These include advances in medical imaging, electronic and telecommunication devices, together with robotic technology and innovative concepts related to highly accomplished operative venues. Economic pressures have, however, brought such highly developed technological methods under great scrutiny with regard to their effectiveness. In the next century, it will be essential to have rigorously applied methods for assessing the impact of new technologies on health care. The assessment stage requires carefully planned measures with the concomitant implementation of stringent protocols to achieve an effective evaluation.

The initial part of this chapter focuses on the development of new groundbreaking medical technology that may become commonplace in the 21st century. The latter part discusses the stages employed in the process of medical technology assessment.

IMAGING TECHNOLOGY

Imaging technology associated with minimally invasive therapy, although perceived as relatively new, is long established and widely utilised in medicine. Radiologists have been using this technology for decades in the form of computed tomography (CT) and more recently magnetic resonance imaging (MRI), providing digital images. This, together with the development of information technology, has led to the current and potential future applications of new imaging modalities.

Image guided surgery can be defined as the use of a radiological tool to guide the performance of an operative procedure. Interventional radiological procedures have gained momentum in the wake of an emphasis on minimally invasive treatment. Magnetic resonance imaging, which does not emit ionising radiation, provides the ideal radiological modality in such interventions. Real time images are obtainable with MRI, where pulse sequences that produce new images every 1.5 seconds provide continuous monitoring of instruments and anatomical planes, allowing for incorporation of surgical procedures to be performed simultaneously. This imaging modality expands the surgeon's field of vision, and will be widely used in the next century to enable a number of procedures to be performed precisely. The development of new MRI systems such as the GE 0.5T Signa SP (see Figure 9.1) which utilises an open magnet with a vertical gap has allowed full access to any part of a patient's anatomy and points the way for the operating theatre of the future. Simultaneous scanning of surrounding structures allows the performance of various procedures while viewing images of the operative field (Gould and Darzi, 1997).

Endoscopic views of body cavities and joints will be combined with corresponding MR images. Interventional procedures performed to date using MRI include real time, image-guided biopsy of abdominal and head and neck neoplasms (Schmidt et al., 1996). Studies have also confirmed the feasibility of performing procedures such as percutaneous biopsies, neurosurgical interventions, dynamic diagnostic musculoskeletal and joint imaging, endoscopic sinus

Figure 9.1: Interventional Magnetic Resonance Scanner (GE 0.5T Signa SP)

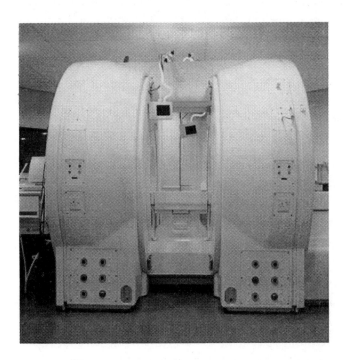

surgery, and excision biopsy of breast lumps. Potential future applications of interventional MRI include performance of oncological surgery, where intra-operative scanning could be used to confirm complete excision of tumours.

Interventional MR scanners will also be used to monitor thermoablative procedures. An example of this application is in laser destruction of malignant tumours, which allows real-time monitoring of tissue destruction with a greater safety margin, thus preventing damage to important nearby structures (Vogl et al., 1995). Thermal destruction can be combined with endoscopic procedures in the accurate placement of laser fibres to the appropriate area (Gould and Darzi, 1997). Minimally invasive vascular interventions will also benefit from MRI which, with the aid of a tip tracking catheter, could accurately detect atherosclerotic luminal narrowings and direct their treatment with percutaneous angioplasties. Three-dimensional computer-aided reconstruction of the vessel will further provide vital information regarding plaque characteristics and treatment effect. Conventional open procedures will also gain advantage from the open configuration of the scanner. Anatomical defects, such as hernias, can be accurately detected during real time dynamic imaging and may eventually be amenable to treatment with injection of tissue glue or cement. In the next century, MRI may be used in a wide range of procedures, producing less invasive means of tissue destruction, and enhancing patient care.

TELEMEDICINE

Telemedicine means practising medicine at a distance with the aid of telecommunications and electronic technology. Developments in telecommunications have been largely made possible by the increasing availability of Integrated Services Digital Network (ISDN), a high quality, all-digital telephone network available in most western countries. Digitisation and data compression capability provides transmission of large amounts of information required for video transmission with less bandwidth or carrying capacity.

Interest in telemedicine as a means of improving health care delivery continues to grow. The transfer of images related to pathology and radiology are examples. This can increase access to high quality medical care from remote, rural or underserved areas. Telemedicine will therefore have a huge effect on the structure of the health system in the 21st century. As well as improving access to treatment, it will act as a force to equalise quality of care.

Real time interactive consultations will be widely used in the next century, such as video conferencing during a surgical procedure, where feedback or guidance is available from a remotely placed surgeon. Interactive video conferencing will be supplemented by a range of peripheral devices such as electronic stethoscopes, monitoring devices, endoscopes and some form of document imaging camera that may be useful for text based information. Dual display screens will be used to show operative pictures on one screen and real time monitoring data, such as an electrocardiograph or electroencephalogram on the other. The alternative form of telemedicine is in a store and forward system, which allows static or video images to be recorded in a data storage device, which can then be retrieved at the clinician's convenience. Radiology, pathology and dermatology are examples of medical subspecialties that will utilise this form of consultation.

In the 21st century, remote consultation may become common-place. Where diagnostic features are provided by images, as in the aforementioned specialities, expert opinion will be obtained in an expedient manner. As well as offering opportunities for real time long-distance collaboration in the surgical field, telesurgical consul-tation will provide a valuable backup system to treat unexpected or complex problems that may be encountered during an operative pro-cedure (Cherriff et al., 1996).

Workstations for image transmission will be a common feature in the workplace of physicians. Junior trainees in a hospital setting will obtain vital assistance and advice in an emergency setting from their consultants or specialist referral centres. Health care workers could gain educational benefits from such a system through feedback of live teleconsultations, which will ultimately lead to a greater in-volvement with patients in the community and a higher level of job satisfaction. This also paves the way for continuing medical educa-tion (CME) through telemedicine for referring general practitioners. Cost-effectiveness of a telemedicine system will require assessment, even though advances in technology may be expected to decrease the cost and advance the scope of such services. The unique medico-legal issues associated with this form of consultation, which may involve crossing international boundaries, will unfold with time. These fac-tors will have to be addressed, together with the possibility of a greater demand for specialist referral from patients, which may ulti-mately burden the health care provision.

ROBOTICS

Robotic technology, which has been successfully utilised by industry, will encroach onto the surgical field. Significant advantages provided by robots include efficient, precise and untiring movements that may be used in a variety of medical applications. Robotic arm technolo-gies, the latest of which are voice-activated, will be used to diminish the personnel requirement in the operating theatre. Complex tasks such as endoscopic suturing will be improved by robotic devices through the restoration of full instrumental dexterity. The voice control mode will also be extended to the primary surgeon, allowing him or her to activate and control all the electronic and medical devices in the operating theatre in what is termed the "intelligent" operating room (Wang, 1997).

Allied to robotic technology is telepresence surgery, which involves operating on a patient at a distant location. Telepresence will add multisensory input from the remote environment to the human operator to create the perception that the operator is physically present at the remote location by using high-fidelity visual, audio and tactile stimuli (Bowersox et al., 1996). The surgeon in telepresence surgery works on real tissues from a remote site where the link is established by an electronic network. Stereoscopic vision, sensory feedback with natural hand and eye co-ordination are features of a telepresence prototype which has developed in the United States recently, consisting of two components: the surgeon's workstation and the operating site. The system has been used to good effect in common operative procedures such as cholecystectomy, small bowel anastomosis and arterial wall repair in the animal model, highlighting the potential practical application of this technological invention in humans (Bowersox et al., 1996). This form of technology could have a significant impact in areas where specialist care is unavailable, such as in small hospitals.

Another distinct application of the laparoscopic telepresence system is "telementoring", where an experienced surgeon at the remote site acts as a preceptor to a less experienced surgeon at the primary site. The surgeon at the remote site has control of the laparoscope and robotic arm, as well as a telestrator for video illustration purposes.

VIRTUAL REALITY

Virtual reality, a revolutionary field of computer ingenuity, will make a major impact in the medical arena. Virtual reality systems create "visual immersion" by generating three-dimensional images that appear to be natural and move in a realistic manner. Skill acquisition will be removed from the operating theatre into a virtual reality laboratory for surgeons to practise their skill. By utilising data from radiological images obtained through computed tomography or magnetic resonance imaging with the aid of computer technology, a surgeon could remodel the relevant structural anatomy of a patient. A planned execution of a procedure based on virtual or simulated surgery prior to challenging or difficult cases could then be performed. Similarly, a radiologist can practise accurately to place a percutaneous biopsy needle or locate a radiotherapy beam following visualisation of a tumour within the patient from reconstructed 3-D images of specialised scans.

Another use of virtual reality in medicine will be in rehabilitating and empowering individuals with disabilities (Greenleaf and Tovar, 1994). Also, virtual environments are ideal for training or educational purposes through reinforcement of information by graphical or visual representation. As this technology progresses, entire surgical procedures will be taught on a projectable, palpable hologram derived from digitised imaging data such as CT and MRI. The future of medical education will ultimately be via simulation and virtual reality.

There is little doubt that technological innovation has propelled medicine into a new dimension, enabling significant progress in patient care. Technological advances will continue to develop new minimally invasive procedures in close association with products that have benefited from electronic and engineering ingenuity. Rapid changes in the practice of medicine and surgery have been evident in the 1990s. Its future development requires a hospital or a medical unit that is capable of supporting and running such advanced technological tools. Bureaucracy and finance may be the key factors that determine the overall progress that such innovations eventually make into everyday medical practice.

ASSESSMENT PROCESS

The preceding examples have highlighted the need for vigorous medical technology assessment in the next century. The criteria used for the mode of assessment have been upgraded in recent years in an attempt to justify its implementation in the public health sector (Fuchs and Garber, 1990). We must not only assess particular instruments, but also evaluate the effectiveness and efficiency of the processes for which they are used.

Apart from its basic scientific ground roots, the continued expansion of health technology assessment requires close interaction with health policy-makers. Medical technology evolves through several stages before its final utilisation, interlacing information on technical aspect, feasibility, safety, efficacy, efficiency and ethical factors. The evaluation process will be a continuing exercise, as new technological developments seek to modify or replace existing technology. Cost analysis and broad-based clinical studies must be performed simultaneously and it is vital that the assessment process incorporates proper selection of equipment or technological tools with the application of suitable predictive studies. The general stages involved in the development of medical technology are summarised below (Murphy, 1991):

- Invention

- Evaluation of safety and efficacy

- Implementation

- Marketing

- General evaluation including long-term effects

- Comparison to existing technology

- Modification

- Replacement.

A multitude of studies or methods will be used in the assessment process. Some of the more common types of studies utilised in technology assessment today are highlighted below:

- Randomised controlled trial

- Case control study

- Cross-sectional study

- Cohort

- Systematic review (e.g. meta-analysis)

- Outcome studies

- Group judgement (e.g. opinion surveys).

Randomised controlled trials offer the most rigorous approach in assessing medical technology, possessing the capability of applying powerful statistical analysis in evaluating safety and efficacy. There are, however, pitfalls to these "gold standard" means of evaluating effectiveness. They are challenging to conduct, as the timeframe involved in the assessment process is often lengthy and costly. Well-designed protocols are required and ethical considerations frequently impinge onto the boundaries of the study.

The initial phase of the rapid development of laparoscopic cholecystectomy and other modalities of minimally invasive surgery offers a good example where randomised controlled clinical studies were pre-empted. Personal reports and retrospective analysis provided the stimulus for the expansion of laparoscopic cholecystectomy from 1987 onwards. It would have been understandably difficult to apply a randomised controlled trial on such a revolutionary development in surgery once the benefits were known.

Case control or cross-sectional studies are easier to use than randomised controlled trials, because they can be completed relatively quickly. Even though case control studies can identify the causes of a disease and side effects of a specific treatment, they cannot evaluate the effectiveness of an intervention, and this is best suited to randomised controlled trials. For medical technologies used to diagnose rather than treat, such as non-interventional radiological imaging, parameters such as sensitivity, specificity and accuracy are used as means of establishing benefit.

Cohort studies, which can also be described as follow-up studies, require an advanced decision as to what the dependent variable or target outcome will be. The main disadvantages related to cohort studies is the large number of subjects and the lengthy follow-up sometimes required, the latter of which invariably leads to follow-up losses.

A systematic review involves a clearly defined literature search relating to a particular medical technology, where the findings are analysed following quality appraisal of the individual papers. Meta-analysis is an example of a systematic review, which involves combining several studies to answer questions not addressed in single studies. Disadvantages related to this methodology include selection bias caused by inadequate sampling and heterogeneity of the sample studied. Non-reporting of negative results associated with a particular technology may also occur. While systematic reviews remain as the best source of evidence for decision-makers, the variation in the quality of each individual study makes the issue of appraisal an important factor.

Group judgement techniques include consensus conference and opinion surveys, the former of which involves collective decision-making by a panel of experts in that particular field. Subjective opinions may be a relative drawback of this method. Opinion surveys are the result of collective judgements formed by experts who are directly involved with a particular technology, with no interaction present between participants to eliminate bias. These methods are used to define cost-benefit criteria when other data required to do so are insufficient (Murphy, 1991).

A recent trend in the assessment of medical treatment technologies is to replace traditional assessment criteria with outcome studies, where mortality and morbidity statistics are incorporated with the technical details and scientific merit of a procedure or therapy. Included in the overall assessment are issues such as quality of life, patient satisfaction and costs. This method can't, however, be used in diagnostic medical technologies where outcome measures are difficult to measure and quantify. The ideal outcome study is one that employs measures of producing data collection that is complete and accurate and does not rely on an individual practitioner's effort in completing forms.

Cost-effectiveness of an intervention plays a considerable part in determining suitability. Health benefits obtained should be at least similar to existing technologies of equal or lower cost. Such an analysis, however, does not give us the precise information as to how much money should be spent on a respective health effect. A good example of this relates to the use of CT and MRI scans, which are widely used diagnostic technologies, but there is no valid data of their impact on the cost of a given disease. An increase in health care expenditure is clearly a continuing problem that can be ill afforded by western industrialised countries. On the contrary, an excellent service can only be provided when sufficient funds are made available. Assessment of patient satisfaction is also important in determining the quality of a given medical technology. The closely interrelated factors of clinical outcome, physical environment and interpersonal relationships of care will need to be considered in this form of assessment.

The impact of technology assessment appears most easily identifiable as the degree of centralised and systematic decision-making increases. It is clear that health care technology assessment depends on a number of factors, not least hierarchical influences on the health care system. For example, in the United States, activities relating to technology assessment are extremely diverse. Many organisations, including government, professional and corporate bodies, insurance agencies and, increasingly, academic health care institutions, have initiated programmes on health-related technology assessment which include codes of practice guidelines (Battista and Hodge, 1995). A similar practice has been slow to evolve in Western Europe, even though our neighbours, the United Kingdom, have in the last few years developed the National Health Service (NHS) Research and Development Health Technology Assessment Programme. The heightened awareness of the need for better information on health care intervention has been due to the separation of purchasing and providing, as a result of the introduction of internal markets within the NHS. This is of prime importance in aiding decision-making processes when planning for future healthcare services. In Ireland, research information on the costs, effectiveness and broader impact of selected health technologies is needed. It is ultimately the responsibility of the Health Department to initiate such high quality research programmes, which can be aided in their task by agencies such as private health insurance bodies.

CONCLUSIONS

The rapid changes and developments that are becoming evident in the field of medicine have created pressure for widespread provision of technology assessment. For the health service provider, this process is of central importance. Appropriate timing of clinical and economic studies are essential and the assessment process should only be performed on selected technologies. Sustained provision of a given technology can only be justified once rigorous evaluation to confirm its need, economic viability, appropriateness and effectiveness have been performed. Medical progress and changing practices are commonplace and are usually the distorting factor that may alter the primary perception of the health care purchaser who may only be interested in the costs, risks and benefits of a given technology that becomes available to the market.

Those responsible for expenditure in the Irish health care system should remain aware of technological advances and obtain all the information associated with such innovations. These technologies must be systematically evaluated in Ireland. It is only through proper evaluation that technology assessment is capable of making a vital objective contribution to the all-important decision-making process.

References

Battista, R.N. and M.J. Hodge (1995), "The Development of Health Care Technology Assessment", *International Journal of Technology Assessment in Health Care*, Vol. 11, No. 2, pp. 187–300.

Bowersox, J.C., A. Shah, J.F. Jenson, J.W. Hill, P.R. Cordts and P.S. Green (1996), "Vascular Applications of Telepresence Surgery: Initial Feasibility Studies in Swine", *Journal of Vascular Surgery*, Vol. 23, No. 2, pp. 281–7.

Cherriff, A.D., P.G. Schulam, S.G. Docimo, R.G. Moore and L.R. Kavoussi (1996), "Telesurgical Consultation", *Journal of Urology*, Vol. 156, pp. 1391–3.

Fuchs, V.R. and A.M. Garber (1990), "The New Technology Assessment", *New England Journal of Medicine*, Vol. 323, pp. 673–7.

Gould, S.W.T., and A. Darzi (1997), "The Magnetic Resonance Operating Theatre", *British Journal of Surgery*, Vol. 81, pp. 595–7.

Greenleaf, W.I. and M.A. Tovar (1994), "Augmenting Reality in Rehabilitation Medicine", *Artificial Intelligence in Medicine*, Vol. 6, No. 4, pp. 289–99.

Murphy, J.R. (1991), "The Assessment Process: a Microscopic View", *Medical Progress through Technology*, Vol. 17, No. 2, pp. 77–83.

Schmidt, A., A. Melzer, R. Seibel and D. Gronemeyer (1996), "Tomographic Guided Biopsy and Cell Aspiration of Neoplasms", *Minimally Invasive Therapy and Allied Technologies*, Vol. 5, pp. 249–54.

Vogl, T., P. Mullen, R. Hammerstingl, N. Weinhold and M. Mack (1995), "Malignant Liver Tumours Treated with MR Imaging-Guided Laser-Induced Thermotherapy: Technique and Prospective Results", *Radiology*, Vol. 196, pp. 257–65.

Wang, Y. (1997), "Project Hermes: Creation of the 'Intelligent' Operating Room", International Congress on Computers and Robotics in the Operating Room 2000, Santa Barbara, California.

PART THREE

Changing Sectoral Demands

10

DEVELOPMENTS IN THE EPIDEMIOLOGY OF DISEASE IN THE NEXT CENTURY

Joseph Barry

DEFINITION AND SCOPE OF EPIDEMIOLOGY

The word epidemiology is derived from the Greek "demos" meaning people or population and is defined as "the study of the distribution and determinants of health related states or events in specified populations and the application of this study to the control of health problems" (Last, 1988). Applied epidemiology in a health care setting is a component part of health services research. Epidemiology is the basic science of public health practice, which itself is defined as "the science and art of preventing disease, promoting health and prolonging life through organised efforts of society" (Last, 1988).

To date, epidemiology has been a largely quantitative discipline. The two main categories of epidemiological studies are descriptive and analytic studies. Descriptive studies answer the questions "what?" and "how much?". They are the most basic form of epidemiological study and the easiest to carry out. By and large, descriptive studies are based on data sources already available. A criticism of the Irish health services is that they have concentrated on data collection without an ensuing analysis of the data. There is scope within the Irish system to answer basic questions about our health status and the performance of our health services by putting a framework in place for routine analysis of basic data. A recent paper on inequalities in health in 11 European countries commented that more detailed analysis could be made in certain countries, including

Ireland, if data on occupation and employment were routinely analysed (Kunst et al., 1998).

Analytic studies are more complex. New data collection is usually necessary and these studies look at cause and effect and answer the question "why?". The two main types of analytic studies are case control and cohort studies.

CHALLENGES FOR EPIDEMIOLOGY IN 21ST-CENTURY IRELAND

Epidemiology has two principal functions within the health services: to describe more accurately the health status of the population through a variety of studies and study methodologies and to assist in ensuring that the health services perform to their maximum in addressing health issues. The important role of epidemiology in the future of the Irish health services is implicitly recognised by the Department of Health and Children (1998) in their mission statement, as published in the policy document, *Working for Health and Well-being: Strategy Statement 1998–2001*, and quoted earlier in Chapter 1.

Health is closely linked to demographics and the age structure of our population will determine some of the major health issues that will need to be addressed. Policy documents such as *Shaping a Healthier Future* (Department of Health, 1994) have led to a second generation of documents dealing with specific client groups; each of these groups have their own health priorities which will be best served by the application of epidemiological principles.

ADOLESCENTS

Ireland has had the lowest median age and the flattest population curve in the European Community since we joined in 1973. While the high birth rates of the late 1970s and early 1980s have declined, a health priority for the earlier parts of the next century is the large number of adolescents and their attendant health problems. Normal adolescent development is a challenging time for all. Teenagers today are struggling with normal development, as evidenced by younger age of use of illicit drugs (Moran et al., 1997) and the reported increase in suicide in adolescent males.

Another aspect of adolescent health that will present challenges for the new millennium is the rise in the proportion of births to teenage mothers that has occurred over the last ten years. Babies of the first generation of teenage mothers are beginning to reach adolescence now.

Routine data sources are available in relation to treated drug misuse and mental health services and a more rigorous analysis of patterns of health and healthcare utilisation from these data sources should help in identifying areas of major concern where resources should be directed. Of more importance than the health services is the response of the education and youth sectors to the growing number of vulnerable adolescents in the country. Early school-leaving has been shown to be a major determinant of later problems, in particular opiate use, in other countries. There is probably a feeling of relief in most schools when children who are very disruptive fail to attend class on a given day. However, a mechanism needs to be found to encourage and maintain people in school up to the school-leaving age of 15. Data from the Health Research Board suggests that over half of attendees at current drug services left school before the official school-leaving age. A redirection of education resources from third- and second-level to first-level would represent a very worthwhile investment. Within the health sector, there has been some move away from the traditional physically based school health examination to a more psychologically based examination. These trends need to continue, as the majority of health-related problems that school children have are psychological and not physical. Territorial differences between the education sector and the health sector need to be put aside in the development of comprehensive school psychological services.

THE ELDERLY

At the other end of the age spectrum, a major demographic shift is occurring in so far as the number of old and very old people is increasing (see Tony Fahey's Chapter in this volume). This is due to increased life expectancy, general economic advancement and better health services in middle and late middle age. This has implications for the delivery of public services in general and health services in particular. While the number of people living beyond the age of 75 years is increasing, the pool of persons available to care for these on an informal basis is diminishing. Consequently, whereas health care in the past was not necessarily concerned with the social care of the elderly, in that this was done largely within the family, this is no longer the case. The pressure on public health services to provide medium- and long-stay accommodation for the elderly continues to increase. A very large proportion of patients admitted to acute hospitals through casualty departments are elderly dependent persons with social rather than health care needs. The pressures that this is placing on health insurers is becoming more explicit, with major health insurers now looking for community rating to be amended, making it more difficult for elderly persons to get health insurance. While these pressures are explicit within the private health care market, they are obviously implicit with the health care sector and new strategies will be necessary to provide effective and efficient healthcare for the elderly. As health promotion and preventive campaigns increase in effectiveness, the proportion of people surviving to old age will increase.

BALANCE OF CARE

Many Department of Health publications over the past 15 years have stressed the need to get the right balance between primary care, secondary care and tertiary care. Epidemiology and its application have a place in arriving at the correct balance. Outcome studies and evidence-based health care generally should increase the likelihood of health care being provided at the appropriate level, provided that the evidence is acted upon. The move towards more robust health information and evidence as a basis for making decisions should limit the influence of vested interests, from whatever source, in dictating how public health services are delivered.

The balance between public and private health care also needs to be addressed. The Department of Health and Children is currently seeking submissions for a White Paper on private health insurance. The reasons so many people opt for private as opposed to public health care are often concerned with the associated "hotel" benefits of private health care, such as pleasant surroundings, shorter waiting times, no lengthy queues and a greater patient choice in how health care is delivered. In contrast, health outcomes are rarely used as a criterion for making the choice between public and private health care. This should be a matter of concern for health insurers and their customers. Linked to the balancing of public and private health care is the issue of new technology. The application of epidemiology to the evaluation of new technologies should result in better purchasing decisions being made as to the most appropriate technologies and the quantity of same to be used in the Irish health system.

MARGINAL GROUPS

Almost exclusively within the public sector is the health care of marginal groups. How society addresses issues related to minority and marginal groups is a good barometer of that society. Two of the most immediate and publicly visible minority groups in Ireland are travellers and injecting drug users. However, a wider minority group is the growing number of multigenerational unemployed families and their dependants. While the economic expansion of the last number of years has undoubtedly benefited the vast majority of the population, the gaps in income between the affluent, or relatively affluent, many and the deprived few has grown. To what extent this gap in income and other social circumstances leads to a change in health status has not been formally documented in Ireland, but evidence from other countries is that income differentials lead to greater health disparities.

IMMIGRANTS

Historically, Ireland is not a country to which large numbers of non-Irish nationals have immigrated. This has changed and there are now growing numbers of citizens of countries of the developing world who are opting to live in Ireland, in many cases because of the high quality of health care available in the country. Existing health systems have difficulty coping with what is essentially a new phenomenon in Ireland. The crudest method of knowing the number of non-nationals resident in the country is the census. The 1996 census enumerated 29,544 persons whose usual residence was outside the State, of whom 20,654 were residents of another EU country, 4,896 were residents of the USA and the remaining 3,994 were from the rest of the world (Central Statistics Office, 1997). This represented just over 0.1 per cent of the population. In terms of a numerator and a denominator base for health statistics, greater use will need to be made of categorisation of persons by usual country of residence. AIDS statistics and perinatal statistics as currently collected do not take account of changing patterns of health care utilisation by persons not usually resident in the country and interpretation of trends is consequently more complex than formerly. Basic questions, such as whether people come for care, stay or bring their extended families will need to be addressed. Racism is a real issue that will need to be addressed in the delivery of health services and the general interaction between Irish people and non-Irish nationals. Evidence from other countries is that illegal immigrants, in particular, have poorer health status than other immigrants and the general population. Access to services is also generally poor and there are barriers to do with language, culture and the perception of what is important from the point of view of health care. These pressures are generally loaded on other pressures in delivering quality health care to the indigenous population.

POSITIVE HEALTH

Over the past 50 years, knowledge of the causation of disease has been well served by classical epidemiology, where single cause agents of illness such as smoking and various infections have been identified by epidemiological study. With the realisation of the multifactoral nature of most health phenomena, it is likely that in the new millennium epidemiology will work in close conjunction with other disciplines such as health economics, sociology, management and health psychology to advance knowledge of disease and response to disease. Efforts are being made to measure the health of populations from a positive as opposed to a negative (illness) perspective by use of health status indices and questionnaires which are focused on psychological health, physical health, functional health or a combination of all (McDowell and Newell, 1996). This is an attempt to make concrete some of the aspirations of the World Health Organisation's definition of health. The construction, validation, usage and interpretation of these various health status indices are multidisciplinary matters. Because of changes in society and demands from customers of health services to be more involved in decision-making, it is likely there will be an increase in measurement of health as a positive attribute in the coming years. Linked with this should be a commitment to carry out qualitative studies in conjunction with quantitative studies so that more detailed exploration of the reasons why health status is as it is can be elucidated.

ECOLOGICAL EPIDEMIOLOGY

Another reflection of the changing world is the development of ecological epidemiology as an activity in Ireland. Most people with a training in epidemiology in Ireland have graduated from an Anglo-American model with points of reference from the English-speaking world and literature. Epidemiology, in the Latin countries in particular, has identified ecological epidemiology as an important activity and it is one that will become more developed in Ireland in the coming years. What it entails is a synthesis of classical epidemiological methods, social policy analysis, political science and environmental epidemiology — investigating individual, family, community and political factors which give rise to certain health phenomena. It is an activity that is most likely to make a positive contribution when investigating health issues such as drug misuse, violence, crime and suicide, which have their main roots in social structures. This approach can also be used in investigating more straightforward health issues such as the emerging infectious diseases. These include AIDS,

Hepatitis C, and multi-drug-resistant tuberculosis, which are health expressions of social phenomena.

LEGAL AND ETHICAL ISSUES

The Data Protection and Freedom of Information Acts in this country are measures which are being brought in for the protection of individuals against abuse, or potential abuse, by large organisations. The nature of epidemiology is that, by and large, researchers working for large organisations are doing aggregate studies from population perspectives as opposed to from an individual perspective. To enable this population perspective to be gathered, sensitive and very confidential data on individuals need to be collected and analysed. The framework within which this is done will need to be clarified. The issue of consent and ethical approval for epidemiological studies will become more important as individuals and populations assert their rights. The ethical framework for carrying out individual-based studies is not an adequate model for epidemiological or population investigations.

SUMMARY

The world of the 21st century will be different from the world of the 20th century and accordingly epidemiological practice will have to alter to meet that change. Epidemiology also presents an opportunity to influence that change by helping to place health and healthcare phenomena in an appropriate context in a developing globe. There will be different levels of epidemiological practice in different global regions and within the European region. There is potential for epidemiology to play a major part in health developments as they emerge over the coming years.

References

Central Statistics Office (1997), "Usual Residence and Migration, Birthplaces, Census 1996", Vol. 4, Cork: CSO.

Department of Health (1994), *Shaping a Healthier Future: a Strategy for Effective Healthcare in the 1990s*, Dublin: Stationery Office.

Department of Health and Children (1998), *Working for Health and Well-being: Strategy Statement 1998–2001*, Dublin: Stationery Office.

Kunst, A.E., F. Groenhos, J.P. Mackenbach and the EU Working Group on Socio-economic Inequalities in Health (1998), "Occupational Class and Cause Specific Mortality in Middle-aged Men in 11 European Countries: Comparison of Population Based Studies", *British Medical Journal*, Vol. 316, pp. 1636–42.

Last, John M. (ed.) (1988), *A Dictionary of Epidemiology*, Oxford: Oxford University Press.

McDowell, I. and C. Newell (1996), *Measuring Health: a Guide to Rating Scales and Questionnaires*, Second Edition, Oxford: Oxford University Press.

Moran, R., M. O'Brien and P. Duff (1997), *Treated Drug Misuse in the Greater Dublin Area*, National Report 1996, Dublin: The Health Research Board.

Population Ageing, the Elderly and Health Care

Tony Fahey

Introduction[1]

In nearly all parts of the western world, the number of older people is growing rapidly while the population of younger adults and children is becoming smaller, in either relative or absolute terms. It is often assumed that this trend towards population ageing will give rise to serious challenges for the health services, perhaps even to the extent of straining the capacity of health systems in the more severely affected countries to cope. On the other hand, many argue that the impact of changing age structures on the health services has been greatly exaggerated and that demographically induced pressures on those services are slight in comparison with pressures from other factors such as medical price inflation, changing medical technology and the rising expectations of health care consumers.

The Irish case is of particular interest in this context, and the present chapter is concerned with setting out what this interest is. It identifies and explores three aspects of the interrelationship between demographic trends and the health services in Ireland. These can be stated briefly as follows:

1. Almost uniquely among western countries, population ageing is *not* a significant feature of demographic trends in Ireland at pres-

---

[1] This chapter is based largely on research carried out for the National Council for the Elderly, as reported in Fahey (1995) and Fahey and Murray (1994), and for the Combat Poverty Agency, as reported in Fahey and Fitz Gerald (1997).

ent. Irish population structures have been more often characterised by juvenation than ageing since the 1960s. The consequent
trajectory of the Irish population means that while some population ageing will occur in the future, it will be delayed and will be
relatively modest in scale when it arrives.

2. The absence to date of population ageing in Ireland has made
    little difference to the size or structure of the Irish health services.
    Though Irish population trends are highly distinctive in interna-
    tional terms, Irish health services are not — or are distinctive in
    ways which has little or nothing to do with population trends.
    The Irish case thus provides powerful support to those who ar-
    gue that population trends typically have little impact on the
    evolution of the health services.

3. Though the elderly population in Ireland is reasonably small in
    relative terms and is growing at a relatively slow pace, there are
    some aspects of elderly demography which pose challenges to
    the health and social care services and which need to be ad-
    dressed in more sustained and creative ways than have been
    found to date.

We now turn to each of these issues in turn, and in the conclusion of
the chapter will draw out some general points regarding the future
significance of population trends for the health services in Ireland.

POPULATION TRENDS IN IRELAND

The pattern of population ageing now underway in Ireland is
strongly influenced by the distinctive population history from which
present trends have emerged. Most western countries in the late
twentieth century are emerging from a long era of demographic expansion and are entering a new period of possible zero population
growth and rapid population ageing. Ireland, by contrast, is on quite
a different population trajectory. It missed out on the long demographic expansion that occurred in other countries since the mid-
nineteenth century. Instead, it suffered a unique population decline
up to the mid-1960s (which, among other things, meant that by the

standards of other countries at the time, Ireland had a population structure that was top-heavy with older people).

The era of decline came to an end in the mid-1960s with the onset of a period of fertility growth and population recovery. That recovery faltered for a period in the late 1980s as heavy emigration briefly reappeared, but it has revived in the 1990s. Population performance in this era of recovery has been by no means spectacular, but it has been enough to set Irish population trends on a more positive course than at any other time in its modern history.

Figure 11.1 provides an overview of the long-term population performance since 1926, with projections of the likely performance up to 2026.

Figure 11.1: Population by Broad Age Group, 1926–2026

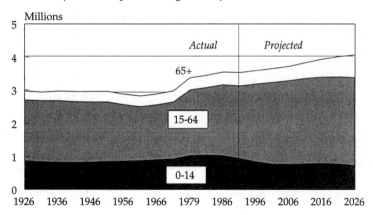

Sources: CSO data diskettes; CSO (1995), M1F1 assumptions.

As this figure shows, demographic decline prior to the 1960s had a particularly damaging character, in that it consisted mainly in a contraction of population in the active-age ranges (due to emigration). The demographic recovery in the 1970s turned that pattern around, in that the active-age ranges showed the greatest growth. The record since the mid-1980s and projections for the coming decades suggest that growth in the numbers of active-age adults will continue to dominate Ireland's demographic performance, to a degree which is unprecedented in Ireland's modern history. Having grown by half a million from 1961 to 1991, the population of 15- to 64-year-olds in Ireland is projected to grow by a further half a million up to 2026, amounting to an increase of almost two-thirds over the whole period. The child population by contrast, having shown strong growth in the 1970s, is projected to decline from the mid-1980s peak of over one million to something of the order of 700,000 by 2026 (the extent of the projected decline depends on the fertility rates one assumes for the future).

It is in the context of this strong overall population performance, and especially the growth in the number of active-age adults, that the nature and extent of population ageing in Ireland should be judged. Figure 11.2 shows that while there has been some growth in absolute numbers of elderly in recent decades, there has been a remarkable stability in the *relative* size of elderly population from 1960 up to the present and for the next decade or so. The elderly are projected to amount to only 11.8 per cent of the population in 2006, little changed from the figure of 11.2 per cent which held in 1961.

After the year 2006, a more rapid growth in the elderly population is projected to occur, both in absolute and relative terms. Numbers are projected to reach around 700,000 by the year 2026, an increase of almost 70 per cent over the present total. Having hovered under 12 per cent of total population for half a century, this growth in numbers will entail an increase in the elderly share of total population to about 17 per cent in 2026.

A further important aspect of the growth in the elderly population is the changing age profile *within* the elderly population itself. The greatest absolute increase is projected to occur among the younger elderly, but the greatest relative increase occurs among the older elderly. Thus, for example, the 65–69 age group is projected to grow by 80,000, compared to less than 40,000 among the 85-and-over age group. However, in relative terms, the increase among the 65–69 age group, at 60 per cent, is only half that among those aged 85 and over, which is 120 per cent.

Figure 11.2: Elderly Population, 1926–2026

Numbers aged 65+

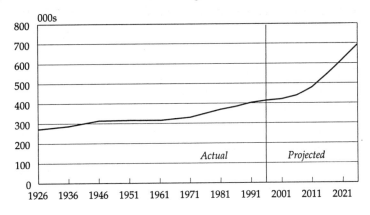

Percent aged 65+

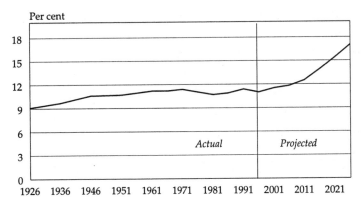

Source: Figure 11.1.

While the post-2006 increases in the elderly and the very elderly populations are substantial, their significance, from a population ageing point of view, is mitigated by two factors. The first is that the elderly share of *total* population is strongly influenced by declines in the numbers of children rather than in the numbers of active age adults. Figure 11.3 demonstrates this by converting the age data in Figure 11.1 into age-dependency ratios. Looking at the *total* age-dependency ratio (children and elderly as a percentage of those aged 15–64), there is a quite pronounced peaking of the trend in the 1960s, and at a very high level. By 1991, total dependency had fallen back to the level of the 1930s and, according to the CSO's projections, it will continue a steep decline until the middle of the next decade. By 2006, the forecast is that, because of sharp falls in the numbers of children combined with growth in the numbers in the active age ranges, total age dependency will be lower than at any time in the present century. Thereafter it will begin to rise again, but the growth will be so modest that by 2026 it is projected to be still well below the levels that prevailed throughout most of the present century.

Figure 11.3: Age Dependency Ratios in Ireland, 1926–2026

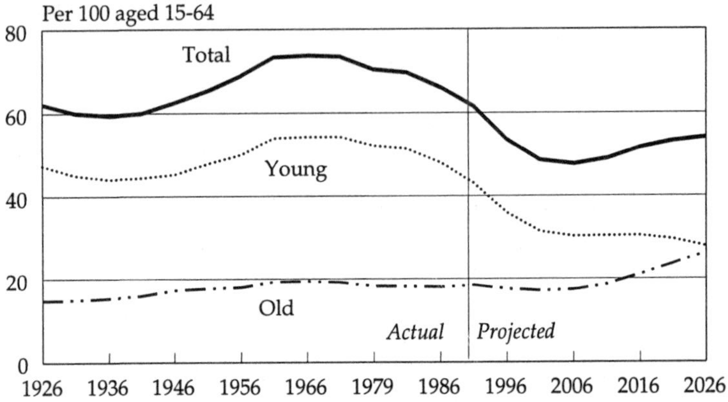

Source: Figure 11.1.

Our particular interest here is in the trend in old dependency. Over the whole period shown in Figure 11.3, that trend is remarkably flat, and indeed shows a slight *downward* movement from the 1960s until the first decade of the next century. A rise in the trend occurs after 2006 but it is quite modest. This overall pattern shows that if the increases in the elderly population shown in Figure 11.2 above are looked at in the context of the growth in the numbers of adults in the active ages, the extent to which they suggest an emerging imbalance in the age structure of the population greatly diminishes.

    A second factor which points up the relative insignificance of population ageing in Ireland over the coming decades is its mildness by international standards. Figure 11.4 gives an indication of Ireland's distinctive international position in this regard by comparing the evolution of Ireland's old dependency ratio over the period 1960 (actual) to 2020 (projected) with that of a number of other European countries. The comparisons show, first, that Ireland had the highest old dependency ratio in 1960 (reflecting the prior history of population contraction in Ireland); second, that Ireland was the only country to show a decline in old dependency between 1960 and 1990; and third, that because of the smallness of the increase in old dependency in Ireland up to 2020, it will by then have the lowest old dependency among western countries. The increase in the old dependency ratio in Ireland over the whole period 1960–2020 (which is about a quarter) is quite slight when compared with the large increases in other countries, which range from two-fold to four-fold. In fact, old dependency in Ireland in 2020 will be lower than it was in the UK, Norway and Sweden in 1990.

Figure 11.4: Old Dependency, Selected Countries, 1960, 1990 and 2020

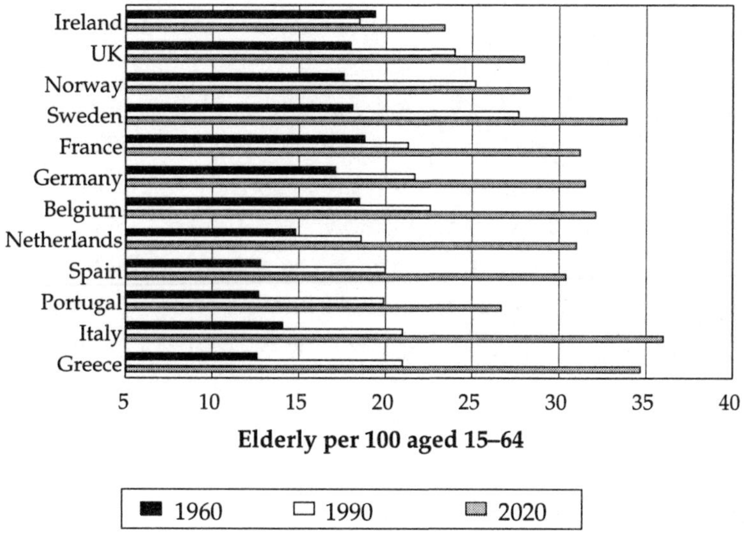

Source: United Nations (1995)

THE IMPACT ON HEALTH SERVICES

The previous section has shown that population ageing has been largely non-existent in Ireland for the past thirty years, will continue to be absent for a further ten years or so and thereafter will begin to occur to an extent that is quite modest by the standards of other western countries. If one were to accept that population ageing is a major source of strain on health services in developed countries, this would lead to the implication that the Irish health services should have an exceptionally easy time of it and should be relieved of some of the main expansionary pressures bearing on the health services in other countries.

The Demographic Non-effect

In fact, there is no evidence that this is so. Despite the favourable and highly distinctive nature of Ireland's present demographic trends, the evolution of its health services has been remarkably *similar* to that of other countries. The same underlying expansionary pressures have been present, the same struggles with cost containment have emerged and the overall shape of the health services appears to be little influenced by the relative youthfulness of the Irish population. Total expenditure on health in Ireland increased fourfold in real terms from the early 1960s to the early 1990s. This rate of increase was generally in line with that experienced in other developed countries. Indeed, for certain sub-periods since 1960, Ireland's health services were somewhat *more* expansionary than the international norm and the health spending cutbacks of the late 1980s served to bring Ireland back into line with international health expenditure norms rather than reduce them below those norms. As far as health expenditure was concerned, there was no evidence of a demographic dividend arising out of the relative juvenation of the population which occurred in Ireland over this period.

A closer look at international experience suggests that we should not be surprised at this result. International data show that health expenditure is not consistently related to any aspect of population structure, not even to such apparently relevant characteristics as the proportion of the population aged 75 and over. An OECD study of the correlates of the health expenditure across developed countries showed that none of the background demographic variables examined, one of which was the proportion of the population aged over 75, had a significant effect, either on overall expenditure on health or on any of the three major sub-areas of health expenditure — hospital in-patient care, ambulatory care or pharmaceuticals (OECD, 1994). In those studies which have shown some effect from demography on any of these areas, the effects are neither strong nor consistent, and sometimes arise more from the proportion of young people than of old people in the population (OECD, 1994). Thus, for example, the United States and Canada are among those countries in the OECD with the youngest populations, yet they have the highest expenditure on health. Though the populations of Japan and Germany have been ageing with exceptional rapidity in recent years, their level of health expenditure remains quite normal by international standards. Greece and Portugal have, in relative terms, larger elderly populations than Ireland, yet they spend a smaller share of national income on health than does Ireland (OECD, 1993).

The absence of a demographic effect is also evident as far as the distribution of health expenditure across care functions is concerned. The division of expenditure across care functions — hospital in-patient, ambulatory medical services, pharmaceuticals, and so on — varies greatly from one country to another and does so in a way that is difficult to relate to any consistent set of factors, least of all demographic ones. Thus, for example, the share of medical consumption represented by hospital in-patient care, in OECD countries in the early 1990s, ranged from lows of around one-third in Japan and Belgium to highs of nearly 60 per cent in Australia and Spain (OECD, 1993, pp. 26–7). There was no parallel variation in population structure, or indeed in any other structural factor that might consistently account for variance in the shape of the health services across national boundaries.

Explaining the Demographic Non-effect

It is counterintuitive that an effect from demographic forces — especially population ageing — on the size and structure of the health services should be so consistently absent. Older people are heavy users of health services. In Ireland, for example, persons aged 65 and over have twice as many GP visits per year as the population as a whole and the usage of health services tends to be particularly high among those aged over 75 (Nolan, 1991). We would therefore expect growth in the numbers of old people to give rise to a strong expansionary pressure on health expenditure — and conversely, we would expect the relative absence of growth in the numbers of older people to have a restraining effect on the growth in health spending.

How can we explain why these expectations are not borne out in practice? A full answer to this question is likely to be complex, but some of the relevant factors can be pointed to briefly here. One possible factor (though it is likely only to have at most minor significance) is that an increase in the number of older people, particularly where that increase is driven by rising life expectancy, does not necessarily entail a decline in the average health status of the population or a consequent rise in underlying health service needs. Epidemiological research is inconclusive on the question of what impact increasing life expectancy has on the total incidence of morbidity among older people, but there is at least a possibility that it entails some delay in the average age at which debilitating illness sets in. We should also recall that health policy in Ireland is committed to achieving real health gain among Irish people. Unless this policy fails completely, we should expect some underlying improvement in population health status to emerge in the years ahead, thus countering to some extent whatever negative health status effects might arise from population ageing.

However, the effect of population ageing on the health status of the population, whether positive or negative, is likely to have little impact on the size of the health services. This is so because modern experience strongly suggests that the dominant influences on the size of health systems are economic and have little to do with either demographic structure or population health status. Across western countries in the last thirty years, growth in health expenditure has been tightly linked to economic growth — the richer a country is, the more it spends on health, irrespective either of its demographic structure or of the health status of its population. In the early 1990s, if one knew the level of per capita spending in a developed country, one could predict its level of spending on health with 98 per cent accuracy (OECD, 1993). This contrasts with the almost total lack of predictive power of demographic trends as far as health expenditure is concerned.

There is no reason to believe that this relationship between economic growth and health expenditure will change in the future. In consequence, although Ireland now is one of the few countries in the western world which does not have a rapidly ageing population, its health expenditures are galloping ahead simply because of its exceptionally high rate of GNP growth. The Government's budget estimates for 1998, for example, provide for a ten per cent increase in spending for the Department of Health and Children, a level of increase which is explicable only by reference to the exceptional rate of economic growth now prevailing in Ireland.

The link between economic growth and health spending suggests that consumption of health services is determined less by "need" in any fundamental sense than by purchasing power. Nations consume health services up to the limit of what they collectively decide they can afford. Collective decisions about the share of national wealth to devote to health care arise not so much from considerations of "need" (since that is such an elastic, indeterminate concept) as from the interplay of powerful forces inside and outside the medical system. These forces include not just popular demand but also doctors and other medical professionals, major commercial agencies (such as drug companies, health insurance companies, manufacturers of medical technology), large health service bureaucracies (both in the private and public sectors), political parties and lobby groups (health issues can provide excellent material for emotive election campaigns). At the limit, one could say that these interests are big and powerful enough to determine that whatever services the health system produces will be consumed — and their tendency is constantly to increase rather than decrease their output. Governments regularly struggle to control these expansionary pressures in health systems, but often with only limited effect.

THE RELEVANCE OF DEMOGRAPHY

So far, the present chapter has suggested that population trends have little bearing on the overall evolution of the health services and, in any event, population change in Ireland at present is more muted and more favourable from a health point of view than in other western countries. This is not to suggest that demographic considerations should be completely ignored in considering the future of health and the health services. In fact, demographic data can be valuable in highlighting those aspects of health need which are important to health service planning. This is most obviously so in relation to mortality data. Mortality rates, particularly when disaggregated in various ways (by cause, age, sex, social class, region, etc.) are a valuable and widely used tool both in identifying areas of particular health service need and in evaluating the impact of existing provision. (As far as the elderly in Ireland are concerned, mortality data suggest that death rates are higher and life expectancies shorter than in most other developed countries, thus highlighting important challenges for health policy in Ireland — see Fahey, 1995.) Likewise, data on the regional spread of population are necessary for planning the regional distribution of health service provision.

In addition to these obvious uses of demographic data for health service planning, there are other less obvious insights relevant to health service provision that can be obtained from the analysis of population trends and structures. For illustration, we can look at one example here — the health implications, particularly for older people, arising from Ireland's peculiar history of low marriage rates in the first half of the present century.

Marriage Avoidance and Elderly Health

One component of Irish demographic decline from the 1840s to the 1960s was a fall in marriage rates and a consequent emergence of large proportions of the population who never married. This pattern of "marriage avoidance" among Irish people reached an extreme in the early part of the present century, especially in the 1930s and 1940s, and remained in place to some degree until the marriage boom of the late 1960s and 1970s. At its worst, this pattern meant that between a quarter and a third of Irish men and women never married, with the proportions of "celibates" being even higher in rural areas.

The legacy of this background is still with us in the 1990s. It takes the form of a uniquely high proportion of elderly people who have never married and are childless, and who have little or no substitute kin to provide them with effective family networks. Figure 11.5 shows that, in the mid-1980s, the rate of singlehood among older people in Ireland was far in excess of that found in any other western country. At that time, 25 per cent of older Irish men and 22 per cent of older Irish women were single. The comparable rates in other countries rarely exceeded ten per cent (the rates of singlehood in Norway and Sweden, which are above or close to ten per cent, are misleadingly high, since they do not take into account the high incidence of informal marriage in Scandinavian countries).

Figure 11.5: Percentage Single among Over-65s, Selected Countries

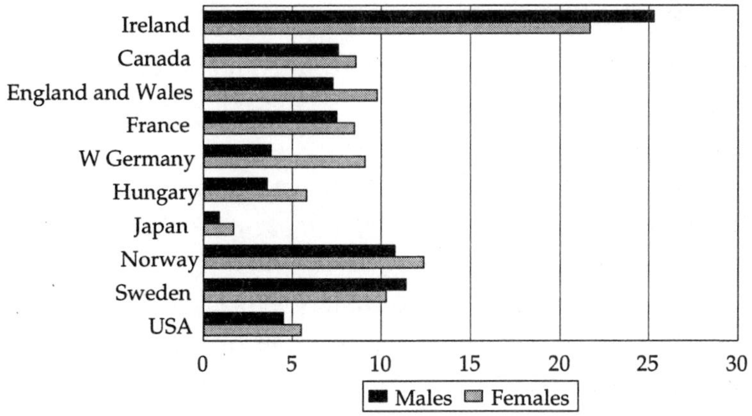

Source: Myers, 1994. Data refer to mid-1980s.

The positive side of this situation is that the rate of singlehood among older people has been declining since a peak of the early 1970s and is likely to do so more sharply in the decades ahead. The decline already evident by 1991 is due to the slight rise in marriage rates which had occurred by the 1950s. However, the dominant influence on trends for the immediate future derives from the marriage surge which occurred in the 1960s and 1970s. This greatly reduced the proportions of young adults remaining single and childless. As these cohorts pass into old age (as is beginning to occur now and will continue into the next century), the elderly population will come to have a more even distribution of family resources and, in particular, will show a decline in the proportion who are without spouses and children. Projections of the elderly population up to 2011 prepared for the

National Council of the Elderly in 1995 forecast that the proportion of elderly men who are single will decline to less than 18 per cent by that year while the corresponding proportion for elderly women will fall to less than 12 per cent (Fahey, 1995: 39–40). These rates of singlehood are still quite high by the standards of other countries, but they are a good deal lower than those of the past in Ireland.

Little attention has been paid to the health implications of these aspects of Irish marriage patterns. These implications fall under two broad headings. One is the effect of low marriage rates on population health. One of the most consistent findings of epidemiological re-search is the relationship between marital status and health — mar-ried people live longer and have better health (both physical and mental) while both partners are alive, partly, it appears, because mar-riage has a protective effect on health (Myers, 1994; Turner and Marino, 1994; Hu and Goldman, 1990). It is quite possible that low marriage rates in the past have been one of the factors contributing to the relatively short life expectancies which now prevail among the older population in Ireland, though it is striking to note that there has been little investigation of this possibility in Ireland.

Another set of implications arising from Ireland's past history of low marriage rates concern the effect of uneven distribution of family resources on the provision of informal social care for older people. It is often said that family support for older people has traditionally been strong in Ireland, even if such traditions may now be weaken-ing. This benign view of the past (and pessimistic view of recent trends) fails to take into account the exceptionally high proportions of older people in Ireland whose family connections are weak or non-existent simply because they never married and never formed fami-lies of their own. In all western countries, including Ireland, spouses and adult children are by far the most important source of social support and informal social care for older people. The high propor-tions of older Irish people who have neither spouses nor children mean that large gaps exist in the usual informal support networks for older people in this country.

These aspects of Ireland's demographic situation are of interest in the present context because they point up a particular health-related need in the older Irish population: namely, the need for substitute means of social support and informal social care to compensate for the inadequate family networks among significant minorities of the elderly in Ireland. Given the extent of this need in Ireland, one might have expected the health care system to have responded creatively to it and to have been particularly inventive in devising systems of community care which would have mimicked as closely as possible the qualities of informal family and neighbourhood care. In fact, little along these lines has happened in Ireland. The traditional solution, rather, has been to rely heavily on institutional care for older people and, indeed, to tolerate a high incidence of social isolation among older people in this country, especially in rural Ireland.

CONCLUSION

Ireland is now in an unusually favourable demographic position, by comparison both with its own past and with the situation in much of the rest of the developed world. Its population has a youthful age profile, and the population dynamics under way at present mean that significant ageing of the population will not emerge for some time and will be comparatively mild even when it does begin. However, if one were to expect as a result that Irish health services would be relieved of some of the pressures bearing down on their counterparts in other countries, one would be disappointed. Ireland's favourable demographic position does not seem to translate into an unpressured life for the health services. There is a remarkable degree of similarity between the general path of development of the health services in Ireland and that of other developed countries, despite the distinctiveness of Ireland's population trends. This leads to the implication that demographic trends have at most only limited bearing on levels of demand or provision in the health services. This implication is borne out by international research. The fundamental lesson is that changes in average consumption rates of health services per person are more important than changes in the numbers of people in determining health service demand. Changes in consumption rates per person, in turn, are determined less by changing "needs" than by increasing purchasing power devoted to health spending, as well as changing patterns of health service provision.

While demographic trends may have only limited value in enabling us to foresee how health systems will evolve, they do have real value in highlighting many aspects of health status and health service needs in the population. The present chapter has pointed to one example, arising from Ireland's distinctive history of low marriage rates and high incidence of marriage avoidance. This history gives rise to influences on health status in Ireland and to needs in health service provision that have not been effectively addressed to date and that point to issues that should be tackled more energetically in the future.

References

Central Statistics Office (1995), *Population and Labour Force Projections 1996–2026*, Dublin: Stationery Office.

Fahey, Tony (1995), *Health and Social Care Implications of Population Ageing in Ireland, 1911–2011*, Dublin: National Council for the Elderly.

Fahey, Tony and Peter Murray (1994), *Health and Autonomy among the Over-65s in Ireland*, Dublin: National Council for the Elderly.

Fahey, Tony and John Fitz Gerald (1997), *Welfare Implications of Demographic Trends*, Dublin: Oak Tree Press in association with the Combat Poverty Agency.

Hu, Yuareng and Noreen Goldman (1990), "Mortality Differentials by Marital Status: an International Comparison", *Demography*, Vol. 27, No. 2.

Myers, George C. (1994), "Marital Status Dynamics at Older Ages", in United Nations, *Ageing and the Family*, New York: United Nations.

Nolan, Brian (1991), *Utilisation and Financing of Health Services in Ireland*, Dublin: Economic and Social Research Institute.

OECD (1993), *OECD Health Systems: Vol. I: Facts and Trends 1960–1991*, Health Policy Studies, No. 3, Paris: OECD.

OECD (1994), "Factors Affecting Health Spending: A Cross-Country Econometric Analysis", Typescript, Working Party No. 1 of the Economic Policy Committee, Paris: OECD.

Turner, R. Jay and Franco Marino (1994), "Social Support and Social Structure: A Descriptive Epidemiology", *Journal of Health and Social Behaviour*, Vol. 35, pp. 193–212.

United Nations (1995), *World Population Prospects: The 1994 Revision*, New York: United Nations.

12

SERVICES FOR DEMENTIA SUFFERERS AND THEIR CARERS: IMPLICATIONS FOR FUTURE DEVELOPMENT

Gregory R.J. Swanwick and *Brian A. Lawlor*

EPIDEMIOLOGY

Dementia is a syndrome caused by disease of the brain, usually of a chronic or progressive nature, in which there is a disturbance of multiple functions including memory, thinking, orientation, comprehension, calculation, learning capacity, language and judgement. These impairments may be accompanied, or preceded, by a deterioration in emotional control, social behaviour or motivation. This syndrome occurs in Alzheimer's disease, cerebrovascular disease and other disorders which affect the brain (World Health Organisation, 1992).

Dementia is predominantly a disorder of older adults, with its incidence and prevalence increasing with age (Ritchie and Kildea, 1995). Approximately five per cent of people aged over 65 years have a dementia while the prevalence of those over 80 years of age is about 20 per cent. In Ireland, the population of those over 65 years is expected to rise by 29.5 per cent between 1991 and 2011 (Keogh and Roche, 1996). The increase in those over 80, the group with highest prevalence of dementia, is expected to be about 66 per cent (Fahey, 1995). In tandem with the rising proportion of older people in the population, there have been changes in family structures which result in reducing the potential pool of carers. Such changes include smaller families and an increasing trend for women to work outside the home.

In summary, over the next decade there will be a dramatic rise in the number of people with dementia, combined with a reduction in the number of carers. The implications of these demographic changes are that the development of specialist services will be required to meet needs for assessment and possibly treatment, while formal support services will need to be greatly expanded to care for sufferers in the community and reduce the burden on family carers.

Policies to Date

For the past three decades, policy for older adults with dementia has been dominated by the principles set out in the *Care of the Aged* Report (Department of Health, 1968). In the 1970s, there was a rapid expansion of health services, improvement in standards of care for the general population, and important developments in both community health services and hospital/institutional care. These developments included the replacement of the dispensary doctor service by the General Medical Service and the appointment of physicians in geriatric medicine. The appointment of a National Council for the Aged in 1981, along with expansion in the departments of geriatric medicine, were of major importance in the 1980s. However, government spending on health care fell significantly in the period 1986–89. In recent years, this trend has been reversed and the first Irish specialist psychiatric services for elderly people have been developed. Against this background, the following policies have emerged.

Care of the Aged Report (Department of Health, 1968)

Prepared by an interdepartmental committee, appointed by the Minister of Health, this was based on the belief that "it is better, and probably much cheaper, to help the aged to live in the community than to provide for them in hospitals or other institutions". It put forward the view that "public and family care should be regarded as complementary — not as alternatives — and that the public authority should endeavour to help the family, not take over from it". These two principles have guided policy ever since.

Planning for the Future (Department of Health, 1984)

The policy recommendation in this report was that

> the majority of persons suffering from dementia should be cared for by the primary care service or by the geriatric service. The current practice of routinely admitting demented patients to psychiatric hospitals should be discontinued. . . . In general, the psychiatric needs of the disabled elderly should be met by the sector team, but, in densely populated areas, consideration should be given to the appointment of a psychiatrist whose main area of expertise would be the psychiatry of old age.

The Years Ahead: A Policy for the Elderly (Working Party on Services for the Elderly, 1988)

This report (hereafter referred to as *The Years Ahead*) defined official government policy for the development of services for older people in Ireland. Policy objectives set out in this report were as follows:

- To maintain elderly people in dignity and independence in their own home;

- To restore those elderly people who become ill or dependent to independence at home;

- To encourage and support the care of the elderly in their own community by family, neighbours and voluntary bodies in every way possible;

- To provide a high quality of hospital and residential care for elderly people when they can no longer be maintained in dignity and independence at home.

Specific recommendations with regard to dementia were as follows:

- "General practitioners and public health nurses should be encouraged to screen elderly people at risk for early signs of dementia; that a panel of people who are willing and available to care for elderly people with dementia be available in each district under supervision of the senior public health nurse to help the elderly person and his or her carers."

- "That day care facilities for the elderly with dementia be provided in each district and that it should be the responsibility of the Co-ordinator of Services for the Elderly to develop such a service, directly by health boards or by agreement with voluntary bodies."

- "That health boards develop day hospitals for the elderly with dementia in the main urban centres, under the direction of psychiatrists with an interest in this field. A norm of two day-hospital places per 1,000 elderly people for the confused elderly . . . be used for planning purposes."

- "That a norm of six beds per 1,000 elderly for welfare accommodation and three beds per 1,000 elderly for high support hostels . . . for the elderly with dementia; health boards provide residential accommodation adapted to the needs of the elderly with dementia as a matter of urgency."

- "That in each community care area a consultant psychiatrist with special responsibility for the smooth functioning of the high support hostel for the elderly with severe dementia and for ensuring that patients benefit from a multidisciplinary approach to their care."

- "As a matter of urgency, that psychiatrists with responsibility for the elderly be appointed in Dublin and Cork . . ."

- "That one of the psychiatrists in the sectors which correspond to a community care area should have responsibility for care of the elderly with severe dementia . . ."

Although not all of these recommendations (e.g. the use of high support hostels) were later shown to be useful, they were influential and based on sound principles. Unfortunately the recommendations were made without indicating how they were to be funded or what services were to be responsible for the different aspects of care and support.

Shaping a Healthier Future (Department of Health, 1994)

This "strategy for effective health care in the 1990s" repeated the objectives set out in *The Years Ahead* and defined the following priorities for older people with dementia:

> "To develop specialist assessment and community support services in each health board for people suffering from dementia, including Alzheimer's disease, and their carers."

> "Strengthening the role of the general practitioner, the public health nurse, the home help and other primary care professionals in supporting older people and their carers who live at home."

> "The target will be to ensure that not less than 90 per cent of those over 75 years of age continue to live at home."

Although the document acknowledges the rise in the number of people in the oldest age groups and that community-based services are not adequately developed, it fails to indicate how these challenges are to be met. In particular, it does not present a specific plan of investment for new or expanded services.

The Years Ahead Report: A Review of the Implementation of its Recommendations (Ruddle et al., 1997)

This report (hereafter referred to as Report No. 48) concludes that "*The Years Ahead* is no longer an adequate blueprint for the development of older people's health and social services". It notes that action in the area of care for older people with mental disorder has been "particularly disappointing" since *The Years Ahead* and that major difficulties with *The Years Ahead* include its non-statutory basis and its significant underestimation of the increase in the population of older people.

Report No. 48 recommends urgent adoption of the Royal College of Psychiatrists' planning norm of one consultant in the psychiatry of old age per 10,000 older people. A training programme for general practitioners and public health nurses to enable them to screen for dementia is also recommended. The report emphasises the need for major investment in all community-care services and identifies an urgent need to increase the supply of beds for dementia sufferers in three areas:

1. Long-stay beds in non-psychiatric settings for dementia without behavioural disturbance;

2. Appropriately designed secure psychiatric units for those with dementia complicated by behavioural disturbance;

3. Beds in geriatric units and hospitals for those with co-existing dementia and physical illness.

The policies as outlined in this section have been based on sound principles and have been influential in the development of dementia services. However, many discrepancies between policy and practice persist and these will be discussed in the next section.

SERVICE ORGANISATION AND CLINICAL RESPONSIBILITY

It is essential that the organisation of services for older people with dementia is clear. In particular, there must be clear guidelines on the responsibilities of, and the relationships between, primary care, psychiatry of old age, general adult psychiatry, acute hospital care, and medicine for the elderly.

Screening/Early Diagnosis

Despite the growing public awareness of the problems presented by dementia, it has been known for some time that general practitioners (GPs) frequently overlook dementing illnesses and that many dementia sufferers do not receive medical attention until an advanced stage (Williamson et al., 1964; Bayer et al., 1987). Based on the false assumption that little can be done for mildly demented patients, most health services concentrate their resources on intervening in crisis situations. Unfortunately, at such a late stage the prevalence of multiple complications is high and the prognosis is poor (Fraser and Healy, 1986).

It is necessary to make a distinction between very early diagnosis and very early assessment. Very early assessment has benefits for research and for establishing a baseline for individual patients. At present it is not possible to make a very early diagnosis with confidence. However, diagnosis is possible at an earlier stage than is usual at present and has direct benefits for sufferers and their families.

If a potentially reversible cause (e.g. thyroid disease) is identified, the appropriate management can be initiated. However, the associated cognitive impairment may not be reversed unless treatment is initiated at an early stage (Chui, 1996). Given the level of current publicity surrounding Alzheimer's disease, those with subjective memory problems but without a dementing illness (the "worried well") may suffer a significant degree of distress until they attend for assessment. If the clinician is able to exclude a dementia, then the patient can be appropriately reassured. In cases when the patient does have a progressive dementia, it is important to confirm the diagnosis as soon as possible in order to allow frank discussion and appropriate planning. Recently, a growing literature has started to address the issue of revealing the diagnosis to patients with Alzheimer's disease (Drickamer and Lachs, 1992; Rice and Warner, 1994; Maguire et al, 1996). Behind the case for telling are the individual's right to autonomy and the right to influence future financial and health care issues through enduring power of attorney, "living wills" and "advance directives". This can only be achieved if the diagnosis is discussed frankly while the patient remains competent. Finally, in order to obtain maximal benefit from non-pharmacological interventions for behavioural disturbance in dementia, caregivers need to be educated and learn appropriate strategies for the management of day-to-day problems as early as possible. If this process is delayed, it is likely that relationships within the family will become strained and inappropriate strategies, which can be difficult to reverse later, may be initiated.

The costs of early diagnosis fall into two broad categories. Firstly, there is a cost in terms of psychological distress for sufferers and their families when they are given the diagnosis. Similar distress may be caused when it is not possible to make a definitive diagnosis. Secondly, there is a cost in terms of the health service resources necessary to provide a comprehensive service to all those with mild cognitive deficits.

There is no doubt that the level of public education, assessment clinics, support and counselling services, family intervention programmes and ongoing research that would be required to make early diagnosis routinely available and worthwhile would be considerable. It is not known whether the potential benefits in terms of delayed institutionalisation and behavioural complications would make such a service cost-effective. However, it is likely that the development of specific anti-Alzheimer drugs will tip the balance in favour of financial savings from early diagnosis.

Discrepancies between Policy and Practice

Shaping a Healthier Future gives priority to "strengthening the role of the GP, the public health nurse, the home help and other primary care professionals in supporting older people and their carers who live at home". Similarly, *Report No. 48* emphasises the role for primary care professionals in screening for dementia and recommends that the appropriate professional bodies organise training programmes to ensure that this role can be carried out. However, there is no formal structure for screening, no provision within the free medical card scheme for routine assessment of people over 65 years, and no specific guidelines for the diagnosis of dementia in primary care. Although a few GPs may carry out "opportunistic screening" of some of their patients, this is hampered by the failure of individuals and families to report cognitive symptoms, poor availability of local services for specialised investigations, and a nihilistic attitude among some GPs who do not have access to specialised dementia services for ongoing management once the diagnosis is made.

Diagnosis and investigation of specific disorders causing the dementia syndrome usually requires specialist referral (Kelly et al., 1995). Responsibility for this service could appropriately be carried by psychiatry of old age, medicine for the elderly, or neurology services, depending on local resources. Ideally, diagnosis and investigation would involve close liaison between medical, psychiatric, and primary care services. However, for those with mild dementia, without physical illness or behavioural complications, responsibility for more detailed investigation and diagnosis is unclear and may be beyond the present resources of the various specialist services.

The "memory clinic", with close liaison between old age psychiatry and medicine for the elderly, provides an alternative service model which has a proven track record (Swanwick et al., 1996). The objectives of this approach are fourfold. First, to identify and treat any reversible causes of cognitive impairment. Second, to forestall deterioration and maximise the potential of dementia sufferers through pharmacological interventions where indicated and, more importantly, by educating carers with regard to non-pharmacological strategies for the management of the dementia sufferer. Third, to evaluate new therapeutic approaches in the treatment of mild dementia; and fourth, to reassure the "worried well" (those without morbid deficits who are, nevertheless, worried about their memory).

At present, only one such clinic exists and it is unlikely that memory clinics could be developed for every community care area. A more realistic approach for the Eastern Health Board (EHB) might be one memory clinic for each of the three areas proposed for the Eastern Regional Health Authority. The EHB Review of Services for the Elderly and Four-Year Action Plan 1995–98 (Eastern Health Board, 1995) proposes three "departments" of psychiatry of old age, each with three consultants. Thus, resources from three psychiatry of old age teams plus the corresponding medicine for the elderly teams could be shared to develop a memory clinic in each "department". This could help to avoid potential problems of centralised memory clinics for larger catchment areas (whereby an individual might be managed in a memory clinic early in the course of the illness but then, some months or years later, need specific services from a consultant-led team which was not previously involved in that individual's care). A modified version of this model might be developed for other health boards with larger rural components.

The Years Ahead recommended "that the function of co-ordinating services for the elderly in each district should be the responsibility of a district liaison nurse". Similarly, the function of liaison between medical, psychiatric, and primary care services for dementia sufferers and their carers could be carried out by a nurse based at the "area memory clinic".

Treatment of Behavioural Complications

The majority of patients with dementia are cared for in the community by families or friends (Alessi, 1991). Disruptive behaviours often result in reduced quality of life for the patient, increased carer burden, and detrimental effects on interpersonal relationships. Failure to cope with behavioural symptoms often precipitates institutionalisation (Teri et al., 1988; Roper et al., 1991). A review of nursing home surveys reported a mean prevalence of disruptive behaviour of 42.8 per cent (Beck et al., 1991), while the available data suggests that, overall, approximately 70 to 80 per cent of patients with dementia have behavioural disturbance in some form during the course of their illness (Wragg and Jeste, 1988).

Dementia sufferers with behavioural or psychological problems are appropriately dealt with by psychiatry of old age services. Domicillary assessment has been described as the lynchpin of old age psychiatry services (The Royal College of Psychiatrists Irish Division, 1998) and has particular advantages for patients with dementia. Firstly, it allows a more valid assessment of the mental state of such patients in their own environment. It also ensures that assessment is provided in cases where the patient is often reluctant or unable to attend for outpatient psychiatric assessment. Finally, it enables a comprehensive assessment of the person's social and psychiatric status, including interviews with other people involved in the patient's care.

The day-hospital plays an invaluable role in the management of behavioural problems, as it can provide a rapid response to referral and can avoid the need for in-patient care. The day-hospital should be situated on a general hospital campus so that physical screening can be carried out efficiently. In thinly populated rural areas, a mobile day-hospital model, whereby particular days are spent in different locations, perhaps picking up patients as it travels to each location, may be a more feasible method of providing this service. For cases where behavioural problems persist, regular respite admissions are essential to enable caregivers to continue care in the community. In combination with psychiatry of old age services, day care, carer support, respite care, and the home help-meals-care attendant scheme play a pivotal role in the management of behavioural disturbance in dementia (see below). Finally, long-stay hospital care should be restricted to the most frail or disturbed patients for whom no alternative is appropriate (Royal College of Physicians of London and The Royal College of Psychiatrists, 1989) (see below).

Discrepancies between Policy and Practice

Recommended psychiatry of old age resources for patients with dementia include the following (per 10,000 population aged 65 years and over) (Royal College of Physicians of London and The Royal College of Psychiatrists, 1989; The Royal College of Psychiatrists, 1995): one consultant, two to three community psychiatric nurses, a minimum of one non-consultant doctor per consultant, one occupational therapist, 0.5 psychologist, one acute bed for investigation/assessment of dementia, 16–20 day hospital places for dementia with behavioural disturbance, 30 continuing care places for severe dementia. However, no evaluation of these norms has been carried out in the context of older people with dementia in Ireland (Keogh and Roche, 1996).

At present, only four psychiatry of old age services exist (three in Dublin and one in Limerick) and, in general, special interest posts in the psychiatry of old age have been found to be an unsatisfactory method of service delivery for older people. This is because special interest posts mean that personnel become overly involved with the general adult component where problems tend to be more robust in their presentation, more chronic, and where sufferers have greater numbers of advocates to support them (Royal College of Psychiatrists Irish Division, 1998). The obvious implication of these factors and the targets of current health policy is an urgent need for major investment in the development of psychiatry of old age services.

Treatment of Concomitant Medical/Surgical Problems

The overlap between physical and mental illness in this patient group means that many require help from both "medical" and "psychiatric" services. Unfortunately, as pointed out by the *Joint Report of the Royal College of Physicians and The Royal College of Psychiatrists on Care of Elderly People with Mental Illness* (1989):

> disparate evolution and resourcing of the two specialities and the "protectionism" generated by the scarcity of beds often led to the polarisation of concepts of the "geriatric" and "psychogeriatric" patient, with each department holding clear views about the type of patient which it would, and would not treat. Where one speciality was better resourced or more responsive than the other, it tended to attract more "inappropriate cases" which might be a cause for pride, but equally a bone of contention.

Discrepancies between Policy and Practice

Delirium is a medical problem, even when it occurs in a person with dementia, and requires treatment in an appropriate medical or surgical setting, depending on the underlying cause. *Report No. 48* emphasises the need for major investment in beds in geriatric units and hospitals for those with co-existing dementia and physical illness. Access for older adults with dementia to appropriate facilities for treatment of physical illness is limited by a lack of rooms in general hospitals and geriatric units where the demented patient can be managed without disrupting the care of other inpatients or being at risk from wandering/falling, etc. Equity of service, as proposed in *Shaping a Healthier Future*, implies that such facilities and appropriate levels of staffing must be urgently developed.

Specific Treatments

The availability of acetylcholinesterase inhibitors for the treatment of Alzheimer's disease raises a number of clinical and ethical questions.

For example, who should be offered treatment and by whom? On what basis are the complex decisions about initiating, monitoring, and discontinuing treatment to be made? Many of the guidelines published in an attempt to tackle these questions lack either clinical or scientific validity. It has been recommended that cholinesterase inhibitors should be initiated on a specialist basis (Old Age Psychiatry, Geriatric Medicine, Neurology) (The Royal College of Psychiatrists, 1997; Lovestone et al., 1997). This would mean that specialists would be required to evaluate more patients with mild cognitive impairment. If specialists are to respond to the expected increase in numbers of patients coming forward and the consequent rise in referral from primary care, additional resources may need to be put in place to deal with this clinical demand.

Discrepancies between Policy and Practice

The first acetylcholinesterase inhibitor available in Ireland was launched in January 1998 and as yet there are no published policies with regard to such drugs. Against this background, a model, whereby specialist monitoring using formal cognitive or functional tests is neither appropriate nor necessary to determine whether an individual patient should continue or stop treatment, would be realistic. The primary care physician should refer potentially suitable patients for specialist assessment to confirm the diagnosis. He/she should then initiate, monitor, and discontinue treatment based on the establishment of realistic treatment goals agreed with the patient/carer at the outset. Ultimately, the decision to initiate and continue/stop treatment will be patient-, family- and consumer-led.

Services for Sufferers of Early Onset Dementia and Their Carers

The prevalence of dementia in the 45- to 64-year-old age group is not insignificant, with a reported point prevalence of 34.6 per 100,000 for presenile Alzheimer's disease (PSAD) (Newens et al., 1993) and 45 per 100,000 for moderate to severe PSAD and vascular dementia (Freyne et al., 1997). A recent Irish study of this group revealed that their carers were more stressed than carers of older dementia sufferers (Freyne et al., 1997). The lack of defined services for early onset dementia sufferers may contribute towards this burden.

Discrepancies between Policies and Practice

The principle of equity implies that younger patients and their carers would have access to the same level of services available to the elderly. At present this is not the case. Diagnosis is usually made by general physicians or neurologists who do not have access to the necessary resources for ongoing care, as these facilities are often accessed only through geriatricians or old age psychiatrists. One possibility is that assessment could be carried out at regional clinics as already described above for the diagnosis of mild dementia in the elderly.

Given their expertise in the management of dementia in the elderly, multidisciplinary psychiatry of old age teams are best qualified to provide on-going care for early onset dementia sufferers with behavioural problems. Although the numbers of sufferers in each psychiatry of old age catchment area are not large (12 identified in the St James's Hospital catchment area (Freyne et al., 1997)), these services are currently operating at full capacity. Furthermore, it is difficult to anticipate resource requirements for early onset dementia sufferers, as this has not been studied in Ireland. However, a guarantee at Department of Health and Children and Health Board level to provide additional and adequate resources could allow old age psychiatrists to incorporate care for these patients and carers into their dementia services.

Carer Support, Home Help, Day Care, Respite Care

Three main types of support which carers would wish from the state have been identified. These are direct payment for caring services, information, and relief care (O'Shea and Hughes, 1994). Services which have been developed since the 1970 Health Act do not have a statutory basis. This has led to anomalies where services are provided on a discretionary basis with geographical variation in availability, eligibility and charges. These services relate directly to the three types of support that carers want and include meals on wheels, day care, respite care, paramedical services, and sheltered housing. The National Council for Ageing and Older People has proposed that such "core services" should be underpinned by legislation and statutory funding (Ruddle et al., 1997).

Discrepancies between Policy and Practice

The current payment through the Carer's Allowance Scheme is strictly means-tested and was received by less than 9,000 carers in 1996, which is only one quarter of full-time carers (Ruddle et al., 1997). A review of this allowance is currently being undertaken and the National Council on Ageing and Older People suggests that a "Constant Care Attendance Allowance would be a fairer alternative". Similarly, Blackwell et al. (1992) suggested that a direct payment for caring would relieve financial stress and confer status on carers as a valuable resource.

Report No. 48 draws particular attention to the lack of a social work service for older people in Ireland. It recommends that such a service should have responsibility for providing support and advice to carers of dementia sufferers, as the social and psychological strains on these carers are well established and would benefit from the particular skills of social workers. They would also have responsibility for advising on entitlements for social welfare, housing, and health/social care services. Social workers point out that the view of social work in *The Years Ahead* is narrow. However, the development of an adequate social work service for older people with dementia and their carers will require the commitment of the health boards and the Department of Health and Children and the allocation of additional resources (Ruddle et al., 1997). In the absence of resources to carry out such an information service, at present this function is carried out by voluntary organisations such as the Alzheimer's Society and the National Carer's Association and through support groups for carers organised by the health boards (e.g. EHB) or the psychiatry of old age services. An extension of this information-based type of service are behavioural intervention programmes for carers. One such programme is currently under evaluation in one of the Dublin psychiatry of old age services (Lawlor et al, 1997).

Finally, relief care may be delivered through day care, help at home, and respite care. Day care may provide an appropriately stimulating and safe environment for the sufferer and respite for the carer. Thus, the contribution of day centres is evident in the social gain for both sufferers and carers, a key objective of *Shaping a Healthier Future*. As already noted, *The Years Ahead* recommended that day-care facilities for the elderly with dementia be provided in each district and that it should be the responsibility of the Co-ordinator of Services for the Elderly to develop such a service, directly by health boards or by agreement with voluntary bodies. However, the status of day care for older people in Ireland is characterised by a lack of dedicated places for dementia sufferers. Where dedicated day-care places/care assistants are available, they are largely provided by the invaluable contribution of voluntary organisations such as the Alzheimer's Society and the National Carer's Association. For the future, several health boards have plans to provide dedicated day-care places and, for example, the EHB acknowledge the "need to develop locally available day care services for dementia sufferers and to expand home support services particularly home care attendants" (Eastern Health Board, 1995: 73).

It is also the EHB's stated intention to expand the scope of the home help and meals scheme "to meet the increasing needs as they arise". However, District Liaison nurses in other health boards rate the service provided as either inadequate or fairly adequate. Furthermore, there is a lack of consensus at health board level with regard to the scope of the service and the level of training necessary. Against this uncertain background, the most recent report of the National Council on Ageing and Older People emphasises the importance of ensuring that the future of the home help service is safeguarded. It also draws attention to the need for improved day care, particularly in areas without a well-developed voluntary sector, improved transport to day-care facilities, and a "particular need" for special day-care units for older people with dementia.

The benefits of respite admissions was recognised in *The Years Ahead*, and this facility has proved to be of "immense social gain to both relatives and patients". Respite care provides support while the usual carers are on holidays or subject to crises such as illness or death. Regular respite may also enable a carer to continue providing care at home despite ongoing behavioural disturbance which has not been amenable to treatment. Respite facilities are available through health board hospitals/homes, the voluntary sector, and the private sector and will continue to be an essential component of dementia services, enabling patients to remain longer in their own homes.

Long-term Care

Two basic concerns with regard to long-term care have been identified. The first is to ensure that people who need expert care receive it and the second is to ensure that arrangements for long-term care are sufficient to guarantee that patients with these needs do not block acute inpatient facilities or put excessive burdens on community-based services. This "poisoned chalice" has been the cause of debate and splits within and between the specialities involved. Furthermore it has led to discrimination against older people with dementia and coexistent physical illness as acute services are slow to admit these patients for acute inpatient care in the absence of sufficient step-down facilities/long-term care.

Discrepancies between Policies and Practice

In early November 1997, three of the Dublin general hospitals had a total of 118 beds being used for patients who would have been more appropriately placed in step-down facilities. The majority of these patients were elderly, many with dementia. As already noted, *Report No. 48* emphasises an urgent need to increase the supply of beds (long-term beds, secure beds for dementia with behavioural disturbance, appropriate acute inpatient beds for coexistent dementia and physical illness) for dementia sufferers.

A draft consensus statement on continuing care for older adults with psychiatric disorder includes the following points:

- Continuing care beds under the medical supervision of a consultant are an essential component of the system;

- Despite full assessment and support at home and in other settings, a small proportion of patients will require continuing care in units staffed by psychiatric nurses and other disciplines under the medical care of consultants in old age psychiatry;

- Good units will usually include no more than 20 beds, mostly or all in single rooms with an adequate choice of day spaces and protected garden, will be local to the patient's home, and will offer respite and day care.

The EHB is currently developing Community Units for the Elderly with four modules planned for each unit providing for the physically infirm, people with dementia, respite care and day care. The units are to be developed to serve particular catchment areas, which would enable patients to remain integrated with their communities. This is a significant advance on previous models using large geriatric hospitals or asylums and is more in keeping with the draft consensus statement on continuing care. Taking a pragmatic approach, within the various health boards, the provision of long-term care will require a review of all long-stay facilities, designating a certain number of places for dementia with behavioural disturbance, ensuring equality of access, and using private beds funded by nursing home grants where appropriate.

Research

Discrepancies between Policies and Practice

Despite the requirement in *Planning for the Future* for accountability and demonstration of health and social gain, there is no information on the incidence of dementia in Ireland and the norms for resources are based on United Kingdom data. On a more positive note, there are prevalence data for dementia and some new models of service have been systematically evaluated from the outset, e.g. family intervention at the time of diagnosis, carer intervention programmes. Other relevant service issues around early diagnosis and how/when to disclose the diagnosis are also the subject of ongoing research. Obviously, this approach will need to be expanded and properly resourced in order to plan systematically for future dementia services in Ireland.

CONCLUSIONS

Equity, a key principle in the 1994 *Health Strategy*, implies that access to health care should be determined by actual need rather than ability to pay or geographical location. Currently, dementia sufferers and their carers do not have equity of access. Particular areas where urgent service development is required include:

- **Psychiatry of Old Age**: Currently only four services are in operation, three in Dublin and one in Limerick. A recent report prepared for Comhairle na nOspidéal by the Irish Division of the Royal College of Psychiatrists recommends that old age psychiatry services be developed in conjunction with geriatric medicine services, with one whole-time equivalent consultant in psychiatry of old age per 100,000 population, assuming ten per cent of the population will be over 65 years. It also strongly recommends that the resource requirements of psychiatry of old age be considered separately from those of general psychiatry (The Royal College of Psychiatrists Irish Division, 1998).

- **Geriatric Medicine**: Over the past decade, the number of consultant posts has increased from 12 to 25. However, not all health board areas are fully covered as yet and many physicians in geriatric medicine are not able to spend all of their time dedicated exclusively to older patients. Given the rise in the number of older people and the demand on resources, more posts need to be filled. Currently, there are clear geographical differences that need to be addressed.

- **Services for coexistent dementia and acute physical disorders**: Rooms in general hospitals and geriatric medicine units, where the demented patient with coexistent physical disorders can be appropriately treated without risk of falling and wandering or disrupting the care of others, are required.

- **Services for early onset dementia sufferers and their carers**: There are no defined statutory services for dementia sufferers under the age of 65 years. Given their expertise in the management of dementia in the elderly, multidisciplinary psychiatry of old age teams are best qualified to provide ongoing care for early onset dementia sufferers with behavioural problems. However, a guarantee at Department of Health and Children and Health Board level to provide additional and adequate resources will be required before psychiatry of old age services can take on this role.

- **Community social work services**: Currently, community social work services are overstretched and concentrate on childcare issues. A social work service for the elderly in Ireland, with responsibility for abuse prevention, carer support, and advice is required to meet policy objectives.

- The recommendations set out in policies to date have not been given a statutory basis and have not been accompanied by an identification of specific funding. If the objectives set out in current policy are to be met, core services, as identified by the National Council for Ageing and Older People, must be underpinned by legislation and/or statutory funding.

References

Alessi, C.A. (1991), "Managing the Behavioral Problems of Dementia in the Home", *Clinics in Geriatric Medicine*, Vol. 7, pp. 787–801.

Bayer, A.J., M.S.J. Pathy and C. Twining (1987), "The Memory Clinic. a New Approach to the Detection of Early Dementia", *Drugs*, Vol. 33, pp. 84–9.

Beck, C., L. Rossby and B. Baldwin (1991), "Correlates of Disruptive Behavior in Cognitively Impaired Elderly Nursing Home Residents", *Archives of Psychiatric Nursing*, Vol. 5, 281–91.

Blackwell, J., E. O'Shea, G. Moane and P. Murray (1992), *Care Provision and Cost Measurement: Dependent Elderly People at Home and in Geriatric Hospitals*, Dublin: Economic and Social Research Institute.

Chui, H.F.K. (1996), "Vitamin B12 Deficiency and Dementia", *International Journal of Geriatric Psychiatry*, Vol. 11, pp. 851–8.

Department of Health (1968), *Care of the Aged Report*, Dublin: Stationery Office.

Department of Health (1984), *Planning for the Future*, Dublin: Stationery Office.

Department of Health (1994), *Shaping a Healthier Future*, Dublin: Stationery Office.

Drickamer, M.A. and M.S. Lachs (1992), "Should Patients with Alzheimer's Disease be told their Diagnosis?", *The New England Journal of Medicine*, Vol. 326, pp. 2947–54.

Eastern Health Board (1995), *Review of Services for the Elderly and Four Year Action Plan 1995–1998*, Dublin: Stationery Office.

Fahey, T. (1995), *Health and Social Care Implications of Population Ageing in Ireland, 1991–2011*, Report Number 42, Dublin: National Council for the Elderly.

Fraser, R.M. and R. Healy (1986), "Psychogeriatric Liaison: a Service to a District General Hospital", *Bulletin of the Royal College of Psychiatrists*, Vol. 10, pp. 312–314.

Freyne, A., N. Kidd and B.A. Lawlor (1997), "Early Onset Dementia — a Catchment Area Study of Prevalence and Clinical Characteristics", Presented at the Irish Division of the Royal College of Psychiatrists, Winter meeting, Dublin, 5 December.

Kelly, C.A., R.J. Harvey, S.J. Stevens, C.G. Nicholl and B.M.N. Pitt (1995), "Specialist Memory Clinics: the Experience at the Hammersmith Hospital", *Facts and Research in Gerontology*, Vol. 1, pp. 21–30.

Keogh, F. and A. Roche (1996), *Mental Disorders in Older Irish People: Incidence, Prevalence and Treatment*, Report Number 45, Dublin: National Council for the Elderly.

Lawlor, B.A., R.F. Coen, C.A. O'Boyle and D. Coakley (1997), "Evaluation of an Education Programme for Carers of Dementia Patients", Presented at the Eighth Congress of the International Psychogeriatric Association, Jerusalem, Israel, 17–22 August.

Lovestone, S., N. Graham and R. Howard (1997), "Guidelines on Drug Treatments for Alzheimer's Disease", *Lancet*, Vol. 350, pp. 232–3.

Maguire, J.P., M. Kirby, R. Coen, D. Coakley, B.A. Lawlor and D. O'Neill (1996), "Family Members' Attitudes toward Telling the Patient with Alzheimer's Disease their Diagnosis", *British Medical Journal*, Vol. 313, pp. 529–30.

Newens, A.J., D. Forster and D.W. Kay (1993), "Clinically Diagnosed Presenile Dementia of the Alzheimer's Type in the Northern Health Region: Ascertainment, Prevalence, Incidence and Survival", *Psychological Medicine*, Vol. 23, pp. 631–44.

O'Shea, E. and J. Hughes (1994), *The Economics and Financing of Long Term Care of the Elderly in Ireland*, Dublin: National Council for the Elderly.

Rice, K. and N. Warner (1994), "Breaking the Bad News: What Do Psychiatrists Tell Patients with Dementia about their Illness?", *International Journal of Geriatric Psychiatry*, Vol. 9, pp. 467–71.

Ritchie, K. and D. Kildea (1995), "Is Senile Dementia 'Age-related' or 'Ageing-related'? Evidence from a Meta-analysis of Dementia Prevalence in the Oldest Old", *Lancet*, Vol. 346, pp. 931–4.

Roper, J.M., J. Shapira and B.L. Chang (1991), "Agitation in the Demented Patient", *Journal of Gerontological Nursing*, Vol. 17, pp. 17–21.

Royal College of Physicians of London and The Royal College of Psychiatrists (1989), *Joint Report of the Royal College of Physicians and the Royal College of Psychiatrists on Care of Elderly People with Mental Illness*, London: Royal College of Physicians of London.

Royal College of Psychiatrists, The (1995), *Consensus Statement on the Assessment and Investigation of an Elderly Person with Suspected Cognitive Impairment by a Specialist Old Age Psychiatry Service*, London: Royal College of Psychiatrists.

Royal College of Psychiatrists, The (1997), "Interim Statement on Anti-dementia Drugs — Implications, Concerns and Policy Proposals", *Psychiatric Bulletin*, Vol. 21, pp. 586–7.

Royal College of Psychiatrists Irish Division, The (1998), *The Future of Psychiatry in Ireland*, Dublin: The Royal College of Psychiatrists Irish Division.

Ruddle, H., F. Donoghue and R. Mulvihill (1997), *The Years Ahead Report: a Review of the Implementation of its Recommendations*, Report Number 48, Dublin: National Council on Ageing and Older People.

Swanwick, G.R.J., R.F. Coen, D. O'Mahony, M. Tully, I. Bruce, F. Buggy, B.A. Lawlor, J.B. Walsh and D. Coakley (1996), "A Memory Clinic for the Assessment of Mild Dementia", *Irish Medical Journal*, Vol. 89, pp. 104–5.

Teri, L., E.B. Larson and B.V. Reifler (1988), "Behavioral Disturbance in Dementia of the Alzheimer's Type", *Journal of the American Geriatric Society*, Vol. 36, pp. 1–6.

Williamson, J., I.H. Stokoe, S. Gray and M. Fisher (1964), "Old People at Home: their Unreported Needs", *Lancet*, Vol. 1, pp. 1117–1147.

World Health Organisation (1992), *ICD-10 Classification of Mental and Behavioural Disorders: Clinical Disorders and Diagnostic Guidelines*, Geneva: World Health Organisation, Division of Mental Health.

Working Party on Services for the Elderly (1988), *The Years Ahead: A Policy for the Elderly*, Dublin: Stationery Office.

Wragg, R.E. and D.V. Jeste (1988), "Neuroleptics and Alternative Treatments. Management of Behavioral Symptoms and Psychosis in Alzheimer's Disease and Related Conditions", *Psychiatric Clinics of North America*, Vol. 11, pp. 195–213.

13

GENERAL PRACTICE DEVELOPMENTS: A PRIMARY CARE-LED IRISH HEALTH SYSTEM?

Andrew W. Murphy[1]

The objective of this chapter is to define general practice, describe general practice in Ireland today within the context of European health care and finally to outline possible future developments.

DEFINITION OF GENERAL PRACTICE

A seminal meeting in the Dutch town of Leeuwenhorst in 1974 produced a working definition of the role of the general practitioner (Box 13.1). Whilst comprehensive, at 204 words in length it does not trip off the tongue easily! Perhaps more digestible is a definition formulated by Barbara Starfield, an American health policy analyst (1994). She refers to a type of care which is first-contact, continuous, comprehensive, co-ordinated and provided to populations undifferentiated by gender, disease or organ system. This is the most elegant and succinct definition of what modern day general practice aspires to.

DESCRIPTION OF IRISH GENERAL PRACTICE TODAY

The structure of the Irish health system, both private and public, has been comprehensively described in Chapter 1. The purpose of this short summary is to highlight those points particularly impacting on general practice.

[1] I am very grateful to Michael Coghlan and Tom O'Dowd for their helpful comments and suggestions.

Box 13.1: The Leeuwenhorst Role of the General Practitioner in Europe

The general practitioner is a medical graduate with specific training to give personal, primary and continuing care to individuals, families and a practice population, irrespective of age, sex and illness; it is the synthesis of these functions which is unique. He will attend his patients in his consulting room and in their homes and sometimes in a clinic or hospital. His aim is to make early diagnoses. He will include and integrate physical, psychological and social factors in his considerations about health and illness. This will be expressed in the care of his patients. He will make an initial decision about every problem which is presented to him as a doctor. He will undertake the continuing management of his patients with chronic, recurrent or terminal illness. Prolonged contact means that he can use repeated opportunities to gather information at a pace appropriate to each patient, and build up a relationship of trust which he can use professionally. He will practice, in co-operation with other colleagues, medical and non-medical. He will know how and when to intervene through treatment, prevention and education, to promote the health of his patients and their families. He will recognise that he also has a professional responsibility to the community.

Eligibility to general practitioner services is dependent on level of income. Those below a defined income level are entitled to all health care services and prescribed, free at the point of contact. About one third of the population are so covered and are termed General Medical Services (GMS) eligible. These patients have the right to choose their general practitioner and are then registered with that general practitioner. They are free to change that choice at will. The remainder ("private patients") pay for general practitioner services and the costs of drugs. Reimbursement of some of the drug costs is available for specific chronic illnesses or when charges exceed £90 in any quarter. Private patients are free to choose their general practitioner, but there is no national registration system to record that choice.

Access to hospital care is usually by referral from general practice, except for patients attending Accident and Emergency services. Other than GMS-eligible patients and private patients referred by their general practitioner, all attenders at A&E Departments are expected to pay £20 per episode of illness or injury. General practitioners therefore perform a "gatekeeping" role in relation to secondary care. However little data exists on how powerful the Irish general practice gatekeeping role is.

General practitioners are private entrepreneurs. For their GMS-eligible patients, they receive a variable capitation payment dependent on the age, sex and geographical location of their patients. There are some payments for fixed items (e.g. suturing) and out-of-hours consultations, but about 90 per cent of GMS income is normally capitation-derived. As a provider of GMS care, they are entitled to a pension, sickness benefit, holiday pay, maternity leave and support for continuing medical education. Private patients pay a fee-for-service.

The Irish College of General Practitioners (ICGP) was established in 1984. Its declared objectives are to encourage, foster and maintain the highest possible standards of care in general practice and to speak on behalf of Irish general practitioners. Approximately 85 per cent of general practitioners are members. Continuing Medical Education is organised by the ICGP through a comprehensive national network of small groups of general practitioners led by local general practitioner tutors.

Profile of Irish General Practice

As there is no central registration of general practitioners, production of a profile of Irish general practice and general practitioners has been problematical. Four important studies have contributed to this area.

The first comprehensive survey was produced by Oliver et al. in 1984. This survey was repeated and expanded by Oliver and Comber in 1994. In both studies, determination of the number of general practitioners was performed by combining lists of doctors registered under the GMS and "mothers-to-be and infants" schemes. This combined list was then checked by local faculties of the Irish College of General Practitioners. A 22 per cent random sample was then drawn from the master list for each health board. The third significant study was by O'Dowd and colleagues on the topic of "Stress and Morale in

General Practice in the Republic of Ireland" in 1995. The ICGP membership list and Irish Medical Directory were concatenated as source lists. A random sample of 900 was then drawn from this total. Finally, the ICGP performed a National General Practice Survey in 1996. Significant effort was expended on establishing a comprehensive database using source listings from (a) membership of the ICGP, (b) GMS doctors not members of the ICGP, (c) private doctors (not GMS and not members of the ICGP) and (d) miscellaneous (advertisement in medical media, etc.).

Table 13.1 illustrates the findings of the three most recent studies regarding the personal and practice characteristics of Irish general practitioners. This is the first time these studies have been explicitly compared. Such comparison is difficult, as each study utilised different questionnaires. Some interpretation has been necessary by the author to facilitate comparison. Blanks in the tables suggest that either the information is not available or not provided in a format which allows direct comparison. There appears to be concordance between the O'Dowd and ICGP studies. Their identification strategy appears to have been more powerful than that used by Oliver. The very large sample size of the ICGP study practically represents a census. It can be concluded that there are approximately 2,500 practising general practitioners in Ireland. Most are male, in their forties, have not been vocationally trained, are working without partners in a non-rural area and serve an average of about 800 GMS and 1,000 private patients from premises which they own.

Table 13.2 describes the workload characteristics of Irish general practitioners, utilising the findings of the first national study of workload in Irish general practice by Comber (1992) together with those of O'Dowd et al. (1997) and the ICGP (1997). These results suggest that the average general practitioner works a total of 80 hours per week, seeing between 130 and 150 patients and participates in a night/weekend rota.

Table 13.1: Personal and Practice Characteristics of Irish General Practitioners (All figures are percentages unless otherwise stated)

	Oliver, 1994	O'Dowd, 1997	ICGP, 1997
Survey Results			
Estimated number of GPs	1,937	2,556	2,427
Actual number of replies	292	753	2,093
Response rate	68	84	86
Personal Characteristics			
Male	85	71	70
Age		<30 yrs: 03	26–35 yrs: 17
		30–39 yrs: 30	36–45 yrs: 37
		40–49 yrs: 39	46–55 yrs: 29
		50–59 yrs: 16	56–65 yrs: 10
		60–69 yrs: 09	66+ yrs: 07
		70+ yrs: 03	
Vocationally trained	22	40	
Working part-time	03	11	13
Practice Characteristics			
Location of practice:			
rural	31	18	
urban	42	44	
mixed	27	38	
Private practice only	09	19	27
Number of partners:			
0 ("Single-handed")	70	51	51
1 partner	20	26	
2 partners	05	15	
>2 partners	05	08	
Working from >1 centre	36	38	
Type of practice premises:			
purpose built	26		
adapted	46		
residence	27		
Ownership of premises:			
personal	69	53	
rented privately	20	19	
health board	11	6	
other	–	22	

	Oliver, 1994	O'Dowd, 1997	ICGP, 1997
Practice nurse employed	15	31	
Size of GMS lists			
average	787	843	
<500	27	29	29
501–1000		39	41
1001–1500		22	22
1501–2000		09	07
>2000		01	01
Size of Private lists			
average	1154		
		<100: 05	None:08
<500		20	28
501–1000		26	28
1001–1500		25	18
1501–2000		13	08
>2000		11	11

*Table 13.2: Workload Characteristics of Irish General Practitioners
(All figures are percentages unless otherwise stated)*

	Comber, 1992	O'Dowd, 1997	ICGP, 1997
Average time per consultation (minutes)	12		
Mean no. of hours	per day		per week
total	12		80
surgeries	03		35
home visits	01		05
practice admin.			04
telephone			03
on-call	08		46
Annual consultation rate for			
all patients	4.5		
GMS patients	6.2		
private patients	3.2		

	Comber, 1992	O'Dowd, 1997	ICGP, 1997
Average number of consultations:			
per hour			5.9
per session			17.8
per week	150		130.7
Consultation outcome:			
prescription	63		
referral	05		
investigation	07		
fixed follow-up	38		
Participation in night/weekend rota		71	
Access to deputising cover		45	
Average weekday rota:			
1 in 1	32	15	
1 in 2		14	
1 in 3		14	
1 in 4		10	
> 1 in 4	28	47	
Average weekend rota:			
1 in 1	17	06	
1 in 2	21	12	
1 in 3	17	17	
1 in 4	15	15	
>1 in 4	30	50	

International Comparisons

It is important to note that comparison of health systems is fraught with methodological and interpretative difficulties. Nevertheless, it is of obvious interest and importance, especially for countries with relatively small populations like Ireland. To place the Irish data in context, Tables 13.3, 13.4 and 13.5 provide comparative figures with four other European countries. Two (Belgium and Germany), according to a categorisation system developed by Starfield (1992) are market-driven health systems, and two (the Netherlands and United

Kingdom) are primary care oriented. Data for this analysis are derived from a study by the Netherlands Institute of Primary Health Care (Boerma et al., 1993). It can be concluded that Ireland, due to the lack of a defined practice population and a mixed fee system, has some market-driven characteristics, but a reasonably strong gatekeeper role. Ireland therefore appears to have an intermediate type of health system.

Table 13.3: Irish General Practice in the Context of European Health Care

Country	Population per GP	GPs as % of All Doctors	Practice Related to a Defined Population	Method of Payment
Belgium	613	46	No	Fee
Germany	1960	18	No	Fee
Netherlands	2325	18	Yes	Capitation
UK	1852	42	Yes	Capitation/ Fee/Allowance
Ireland	1587	42	Yes (for a third)	Capitation/Fee

Table 13.4: The Role of General Practitioners as Gatekeepers in Europe

Country	GP as Gatekeeper	Referrals per 1,000 Patients	Delay from Referral to Specialist Appointment (Days)
Belgium	No	38	7.5
Germany	No	55	6.9
Netherlands	Yes	44	10.8
UK	Yes	47	36.3
Ireland	Yes (generally)	42	27.4

Table 13.5: General Practice Workload in Europe

Country	Direct Encounters per Week	Home Visits as a %	Physician Contacts per Capita per Year	Duration of Encounter in Minutes
Belgium	135	46	7.5	11
Germany	220	16	11.5	?
Netherlands	141	19	5.1	9.1
UK	128	15	4.5	5.8 .
Ireland	135	17	6.6	12

FUTURE DEVELOPMENTS

Prediction is difficult, especially when it comes to the future! I have categorised developments as either, in my view, "inevitable" or "possible".

Inevitable Developments

Changing Demographics

In the first 20 years of the 21st century, significant numbers of general practitioners from the current "bulge" between the ages of 35 and 50 will retire. Their replacements will be young and vocationally trained. The implications of these developments are unclear, but it is probable that the aspirations of such future practitioners regarding both their type of workload and working conditions will be significantly different from those of their predecessors.

The numbers of females completing both undergraduate medical education and general practice postgraduate vocational schemes will continue to be well in excess of 50 per cent. However, as shown by the work of Oliver and Comber (1994) and Bradley et al. (1996), women, in comparison to their male counterparts, are much less likely to remain in general practice or achieve the status of principal. The present oversupply of vocationally trained general practitioners, for the currently limited number of available GMS posts, is a result of the lack of explicit manpower planning for Irish general practice. The loss of female graduates could be construed as a "safety valve" for this situation. This is a short-sighted and unsustainable viewpoint. Explicit manpower planning and development of part-time principalships will be essential for the development of general practice. An expansion of the role of general practice (see below) will also require larger numbers of well-trained graduates.

Chapter 11 in this book extensively describes the implications of the "greying" of Ireland's relatively young population. An increase in the number of older patients will significantly increase practice workload and in some rural areas, should depopulation result, threaten practice viability.

Computerisation

The National Health Strategy (1994), noting the lack of data relating to disease process and morbidity in the community, set the specific aim of having 80 per cent of GMS practices computerised within four years. Certainly, more practices than ever before will have computers. The challenge, however, is to ensure their optimal use, as opposed to being restricted to mere word processing. The present quandary is that computerisation has significant, possibly short-term, workload implications for the general practitioner, benefits the individual patient little in absolute terms, but holds tremendous promise for the care of populations and inter-sectoral exchange of information. The potential of computerisation will only be realised when the minimum dataset required to improve quality of care has been defined and procured. The extra workload for general practitioners in achieving this must be recognised.

Out of Hours Care

The study by O'Dowd et al. (1997) of Irish general practitioners showed that out-of-hours work decreased morale whilst increasing stress. Over two-thirds of UK general practitioners recently voted to opt out of their 24-hour commitment (Hurwitz, 1995). The demands and expectations of patients for out-of-hours care has outstripped many general practitioners' willingness and ability to meet them. In the UK, the use of deputising services and co-operatives is significantly increasing (Hallam, 1994). The latter can be defined as non-commercial organisations, led and staffed by local principals, which enable doctors to spend less time on call by working in a large rota. Similar trends can be expected in Ireland but will be diminished by two important factors. Firstly, private practice is viewed as a powerful disincentive to sharing workload between practices. Secondly, deputising and co-operative services are more difficult to organise in sparsely populated areas. For significant numbers of rural Irish general practitioners, the nature of out-of-hours care is unlikely to change.

Patient Registration

The National Health Strategy (Department of Health, 1994) stated that the "general practice units will seek to introduce a system of patient registration". Steps towards national patient registration are currently occurring in the national immunisation and breast screening programmes. This development is imperative if the important potential of preventive medicine is to be achieved for Irish patients. It is a key target.

Private Health Insurance

Private health insurance presently has a minimal role in Irish primary care. Payment is restricted to a limited list of procedures. The advent of market competition has changed little. This situation can be expected to change, with the role of "gatekeeping" receiving especially close attention.

Possible Developments

Research and Development

The clinical decisions made in primary care are of vital importance to patients and the health services generally; for example, were general practitioners to increase their present referral rates to hospital (at about five per cent of all patients seen) by only ten per cent, the Irish health system would be immediately placed under intolerable pressure. Yet paradoxically, the evidence base for much of the decision-making and interventions in general practice is inadequate.

The importance of the symbiotic relationship in secondary care between high quality patient care and high quality research and development has long been accepted. Research in Irish general practice can presently be perceived as an activity performed by a few consenting adults in the privacy of their own practices. The recent establishment of academic departments of general practice in the five universities, together with work by the Irish College of General Practitioners, is welcome but not sufficient. For a research and development culture to develop in general practice, support from central sources to recruit, develop and retain personnel is required. The Department of Health in the UK has recognised this through the publication of the report *R&D in Primary Care* (1997) and the doubling of annual NHS primary care research funding to £50 million. As much primary care research is health services related, it is especially important for the unique Irish health care system to develop a strong primary care research and development culture. The development of general practice based research networks allied to the universities and the Postgraduate Resource Centre of the Irish College will be an important, but potentially difficult, objective.

Changes to Patient Eligibility

As described earlier, the separatist eligibility status of patients for general practice care contributes to the categorisation of Ireland as having an intermediate type of health system regarding orientation to primary health care. The private/GMS mix is an integral component of the entrepreneurial nature of Irish general practice. Indeed, it is a contractual specification, between doctors and the Department of Health and Children, that GMS eligibility cannot rise above 40 per cent without prior discussion. Modifications regarding eligibility at the extremes of age have been proposed. Accepting that these age groups are relatively frequent consulters (and therefore remunerative in private practice) and that general practice is currently underfunded, strongly infers that such modifications must be undertaken with caution.

Some commentators have suggested a radical review of GMS eligibility, to the point of universal access. This option was comprehensively voted down by an emergency general meeting of the Irish Medical Organisation in 1997. As long as significant numbers of patients attend secondary care privately, it would appear inimical to the development of general practice to be the sole health care provider of universal eligibility. Nevertheless, there may be a certain historical resonance between the result and the first plebiscite of British Medical Association members in 1948 before the introduction of the NHS — doctors initially overwhelmingly opposed it (Timmins, 1995)!

Role of User Fees

The two objectives of user fees are firstly to discourage unnecessary utilisation and secondly to raise revenue. An Irish example is the Health (Outpatient Charges) Regulations, 1994, which were designed to encourage private patients to consult their general practitioner before attending the A&E department. The Regulations specified that a charge of £12 was to be applied to patients who attended without a letter of referral from their general practitioner. The charge was increased to £20 in 1998. It is common for user fees to be a component of separatist health care systems and, with the present clamour for health care efficiency, it is possible that their role may be enlarged.

However, an international review (Creese, 1997) concludes that "as an instrument of health policy, user fees have proved to be blunt and of limited success and to have potentially serious side effects in terms of equity". Nolan (1993), in a comprehensive review referring specifically to Ireland, concurred, stating that "the case for charges is for the most part a weak one . . . [they are] a soft option, alleviating the need to address how to get better value for money in the health services". Indeed, it has been shown that the Health (Outpatient Charges) Regulations, 1994, did not achieve their objective of reducing A&E attendances (Murphy et al., 1997). Whilst user fees may prove politically difficult to resist, it would be unfortunate for such policy-making to ignore the available evidence.

Role of the "Personal Doctor"

McCormick (1996) has stated that:

> the gradual and now considerable erosion of the notion of a personal doctor who has knowledge of patients as people and who has earned their trust has diminished; this is the cause of much that is bad in medicine.

The often-derided high proportion of singlehanded Irish general practitioners may have paradoxically facilitated, for the patient, a sense of trust in their personal doctor and, for the practitioner, a sense of professional autonomy. It will be important to ensure that the developments described above do not contribute to further diminution of this important relationship.

THE NATURE OF GENERAL PRACTICE: A TRULY PRIMARY CARE LED HEALTH SERVICE?

Irish general practitioners can be considered to be overworked but underemployed. A significant volume of work is reactive in nature, dealing with the effects of chronic diseases. In the GMS system, there is little incentive to promote health and utilise preventive health strategies. Private practice may emphasise patient turnover and medical procedures rather than appropriate evidence-based interventions. The relative fragmentation and isolation of primary care results in general practitioners undertaking some work which may have been appropriately performed by other primary care workers such as practice or public health nurses. Some services are predominantly undertaken in hospitals — for example, minor surgery and the monitoring of oral anticoagulants — which are more appropriate to the community setting.

Every system is perfectly designed to achieve the results it achieves (Berwick, 1996). A change in the nature of general practice will only occur with the provision of adequate funding. Fifty per cent of all public health expenditure in Ireland is received by the general hospital programme; 16 per cent by community health (OECD, 1997). Whilst the annual increase in expenditure during the 1990s has been 12 per cent for the latter and nine for the former, such a differential will not stimulate significant primary care development.

The National Health Strategy (Department of Health, 1994), in describing general practitioners as a key ingredient of primary care, lacks ambition. General practitioners can play a pivotal role in *all* the health services of the 21st century — co-ordinating the care of patients, providing specialised advice, treatment, health promotion and care in partnership with other professionals and agencies, and adapting and responding to the needs of local communities. A truly primary care led health service. Significant new investment in primary care — both in personnel and infrastructure — will be necessary for the full potential of each general practice consultation to be realised.

References

Berwick, D.M. (1996), "A Primer on Leading the Improvement of Systems", *British Medical Journal*, Vol. 312, pp. 619–22.

Boerma, W.G.W., F.A.J.M. de Jong and P.H. Mulder (1993), "Health Care and General Practice across Europe", *NIVEL*, Utrecht.

Bradley, F., A.W. Murphy and S. Lamb (1996), "A National Survey of Career Pathways of all Graduates of Vocational Training Programmes in General Practice in Ireland", *European Journal of General Practice*, Vol. 2, pp. 157–61.

Comber, H. (1992), *The First National Study of Workload in General Practice*, Dublin: Irish College of General Practitioners.

Creese, A. (1997), "User Fees" (Editorial), *British Medical Journal*, Vol. 315, pp. 202–3.

Department of Health (1994), *Shaping a Healthier Future: a Strategy for Effective Healthcare in the 1990s*, Dublin: Stationery Office.

Department of Health (UK) (1997), *R&D in Primary Care*, National Working Group Report, London: HMSO.

Hallam, L. (1994), "Primary Medical Care outside Normal Working Hours: Review of Published Work", *British Medical Journal*, Vol. 308, pp. 249–53.

Hurwitz, B. (1995), "The New Out of Hours Agreement for General Practitioners", *British Medical Journal*, Vol. 311, pp. 824–5.

Irish College of General Practitioners (1997), *National General Practice Survey. Section 1: Personal Information*, Dublin: Irish College of General Practitioners.

McCormick, J. (1996), "Death of the Personal Doctor", *Lancet*, Vol. 348, pp. 667–8.

Murphy, A.W., C. Leonard, P.K. Plunkett, G. Bury, F. Lynam, M. Smith and D. Gibney (1997), "Effect of the Introduction of a Financial Incentive for Fee-paying A&E Attenders to Consult their General Practitioner before Attending the A&E Department", *Family Practice*, Vol. 14, pp. 407–10.

Nolan, B. (1993), "Charging for Public Health Services in Ireland: Why and How?", Paper No. 19, Dublin: ESRI.

O'Dowd, T., H. Sinclair and M. McSweeney (1997), *Stress and Morale in General Practice in the Republic of Ireland*, Dublin: Irish College of General Practitioners.

OECD (1997), *OECD Economic Surveys: Ireland*, Paris: Publications Service, OECD, pp. 120 and 131.

Oliver, B., N. Meagher, M. Cole (1984), "The Present State of General Practice in Ireland. Modern Medicine of Ireland" (Suppl) (May).

Oliver, B. and H. Comber (1994), "Changes in the Structure of Irish General Practice over the Past Decade: 1982 to 1992", Dublin: Irish College of General Practitioners.

Starfield, B. (1992), *Primary Care: Concept, Evaluation and Policy*, Oxford: Oxford University Press.

Starfield, B. (1994), "Is Primary Care Essential?" *Lancet*, Vol. 344, pp. 1129–33.

Timmins, N. (1995), *The Five Giants: a Biography of the Welfare State*, London: Harper Collins, p. 130.

14

Nursing in 21st Century Ireland: Opportunities for Transformation

Maeve Dwyer and *Peta Taaffe*

Introduction

Nurses are generally assumed to be the backbone of the health services. Indeed, the prospect of running the service without them would be unthinkable. In Ireland, nurses currently account for 40 per cent of the health services workforce and approximately one-third of health expenditure on salaries.

Historically, nursing in Ireland has been an almost totally female occupation. At the end of 1997, there were a total of 56,155 nurses recorded on the Irish Register of Nurses and of these approximately 66 per cent were eligible to practise. Of the total number of nurses registered at the end of 1997, 94 per cent were women. In the past, Irish student nurses tended to come from a farming (28 per cent) and middle class (40 per cent) background. The 1988 study of all but one of the Irish general nurse training schools found that 97 per cent of students had university entrance level of education (McCarthy, 1988).

Irish society in the 20th century regarded nurses highly, believing them to be in the main a well-motivated and vocationally oriented workforce. Nursing as a career in this country has been distinguished by job security, the belief that nursing is a respected career, the ability to travel with a nursing qualification and the acknowledgement by nurses themselves of the intrinsic worth of what they do.

For many decades, we have been reassured by the belief that Irish nurses are the best in the world. This belief led us to the erroneous deduction that it was the Irish system of nurse training that was responsible. In reality, it was probably due to the Irish personality characteristics of interest in people, warmth and empathy. Irish nursing, for much of the 20th century, had a very complacent attitude with regard to manpower planning, which was non-existent here during a period when the rest of Europe was experiencing shortages of nurses.

Religious orders played a very significant part in the development of Irish nursing (Dwyer, 1983). Hospitals run and managed by religious were generally considered to be among the most prestigious in terms of nurse training. For much of the 20th century, nursing as a career choice in Ireland was regarded as being on a par with the religious life and teaching, being both respected and secure. Nursing's popularity may have been influenced by the fact that nursing students were paid salaries, in contrast to other students.

Members of the public who use any part of the health services meet and relate with nurses. But most people have very little idea of the broad scope of activities in which nurses are involved. Ireland has registered general nurses, psychiatric nurses, midwives, sick children's nurses, public health nurses and nurses of the mentally handicapped. Within each of these categories, nurses have begun to develop a variety of specialist roles. Psychiatric nurses may work as behavioural therapists or community psychiatric nurses. The acute general hospitals have developed the greatest range of nursing specialities. Most large hospitals now employ oncology nurses, diabetic nurses, stoma therapists, intensive care nurses, accident and emergency nurses, anaesthetic and theatre nurses. These specialist roles have contributed to a transformation in nursing which is set to increase exponentially in the 21st century.

AN BORD ALTRANAIS

Nursing in Ireland is regulated by An Bord Altranais (the Irish Nursing Board), under the Nurses' Act, 1985. An Bord Altranais consists of 29 members, 17 of whom are nurses elected by nurses. The remainder are appointed by the Minister for Health. The main functions of An Bord Altranais under the 1985 Nurses' Act relate to:

- The maintenance of a Register of Nurses;

- The control of education and training of nurses;

- The operation of the fitness to practice procedures;

- The ensuring of compliance with European Union Directives on nursing and midwifery.

In order to register as a nurse, a student must pass the registration examinations set by An Bord Altranais. Since 1994, students undertaking college-based diploma programmes also sit an examination set by their college. For nursing and midwifery students, this duplication is problematic, considering that the medical and dental councils accept examination by the university medical and dental schools for registration. Irish nurses have been critical of their regulatory body for its cautious response to change.

Irish nursing is also regulated by directives issued by the European Union. An Bord Altranais is charged with ensuring that Ireland complies with these directives. The purpose of the European directives is to enable general nurses and midwives to practise their profession in any member state. Despite its relatively small geographic size, there is a high degree of diversity in the systems of nursing regulation in Europe. The nature of professional nursing and midwifery practice varies considerably from country to country. The establishment of freedom of movement in the EU has done little to benefit Irish health agencies, since in the past, the pattern of movement has tended to be Irish nurses leaving to work in Europe, rather than the reverse.

As an international regulatory body, it will be the responsibility of An Bord Altranais in the 21st century to develop, extend and strengthen the government-professional partnership. Margretta Styles, President of the International Council of Nurses, has sug-

---

* However, in 1998, the benefit of freedom of movement within the EU was brought home forcefully to Irish health agencies. By August 1998, nurse managers from many of Dublin's large hospitals were actively recruiting (some even using recruiting agencies) in the UK and the Nordic countries of the EU.

gested an appropriate 21st century model for regulatory bodies in nursing. She considers that regulatory bodies in nursing should:

- Go beyond initial assessment to continued assessment, to assure continued competence of nurses and the maintenance of safe practice;

- Ensure the relevance and quality of schools and programmes of nursing education;

- Provide for nurses to demonstrate special, advanced, multiple and cumulative areas of expertise with transferable credentials;

- Be open-ended and dynamic to adapt to the changing needs of the health care environment and the evolving and expanding capabilities of nurses;

- Include a more direct role in credentialing for the profession;

- Serve as an advocate for consumers and for nurses' competence;

- Encourage public participation to promote the development of policies and credentials, enabling consumers to be knowledgeable managers of their own health care (Styles, 1997).

COMMISSION ON NURSING

The rationalisation of hospital services in Ireland at the end of the 1980s led to the emergence of a leaner health service. This had both positive and negative consequences for nurses. On the negative side, nurses frequently took the brunt of public dissatisfaction with the perceived reduction and restriction of services. This caused nurses great stress and strain. The first hint of registered nurse wastage was experienced. On the positive side, such factors as reduced hospital stay, new treatment modalities, resulting from new technology and the increase in day services, created opportunities for some nurses to develop more independent and autonomous specialist roles. The growth in the number and complexity of specialist nurses with greater autonomy is a key ingredient of the transformation in Irish nursing which correlates with changes in the structure and organisation of our health services. Radical remedies have to be applied to curb growth in health care costs. Ireland is one of the few OECD countries that has reduced its share of GNP devoted to health. During the period 1980 to 1993, the fall in our share of GNP devoted to health was approximately 23 per cent. This contrasts with an average 24 per cent increase experienced in 13 other OECD countries over the same period (OECD Economic Surveys, 1997).

In Ireland, the most dramatic changes occurred in the 1980s in the acute hospital sector. It is not without significance that this is the sector in which the greatest nursing transformation can be observed. With the wisdom of hindsight, it is easy to understand why, in 1996, an occupational group known for their institutional loyalty, their strong vocational ethos and with no background or experience of industrial action came to the brink of a national strike. The crisis was avoided by the intervention of the Labour Court. An across-the-board salary increase and the offer to establish a Commission on Nursing defused an incredibly tense situation within hours of the commencement of industrial action.

The Commission on Nursing was established following a recommendation from the Labour Court which recognised that there had been extensive changes in the requirements placed on nurses. The Court suggested that the issues to be considered by the Commission would be wide-ranging. The Minister for Health established the Commission on Nursing on 21 March 1997.

The final report of the Commission will be published in September 1998. Irish nurses hope that, in accordance with its terms of reference, it will provide a secure basis for the further professional development of nursing in the context of anticipated changes in health services, their organisation and delivery.

The most significant factors that will influence the successful transformation of Irish nursing include recruitment, pre-registration and continuing education, retention, specialisation and advanced practice and the management of nursing.

Box 14.1: Commission on Nursing Terms of Reference

The Commission will examine and report on the role of nurses in the health services including:

- The evolving role of nurses, reflecting their professional development and their role in the overall management of services;

- Promotional opportunities and related difficulties;

- Structural and work changes appropriate to the effective and efficient discharge of that role;

- The requirement placed on nurses, both in training and the delivery of services;

- Segmentation of the grade;

- Training and education requirement.

In its recommendations, it should seek to provide a secure basis for further professional development of nursing in the context of anticipated changes in health services, their organisation and delivery.

RECRUITMENT INTO NURSING

For most of the 20th century, Ireland was privileged to have a large pool of highly educated school leavers interested in nursing as a career. It is likely that we will continue to have well-educated potential students in the future. What is less certain is how many of them will choose nursing as a career.

In the 21st century, recruitment into nursing looks set to decline. A 1997 review of recruitment and selection procedures for student nurses paints a gloomy picture:

> The nursing profession in Ireland is likely to have considerable difficulties in future years in filling the training places available in the schools of nursing on its diploma/registration programmes. At a time when the numbers of school leavers coming forward for third level education are falling, the training, education and career opportunities available to them continue to increase. Competition from schools of nursing in Great Britain will add to the difficulty. To meet these com-

petitive pressures an active promotional campaign to stimulate the interest of Irish school leavers in the nursing profession will be necessary (Nursing Applications Centre, 1997).

Up to the 1990s, no serious efforts were made by Irish health agencies
to encourage young people into nursing. Availability of information
about nursing as a career, together with centralisation of recruitment
and selection, should have a positive effect on nursing recruitment,
putting it into the mainstream of third-level education choices. An
Bord Altranais has now produced an information booklet for potential students. Other forms of media will need to be used in the future
in an increasingly competitive recruitment market.

PRE-REGISTRATION EDUCATION

Up to 1994, nurses in Ireland were training in apprenticeship programmes that varied from 36 to 40 months, a maximum of six
months being classroom-based. The training took place entirely in
hospitals with no involvement by third level institutions. This system
of training produced an extremely practical but unquestioning practitioner, institutional patriots with an unswerving loyalty to their
training hospital. Treacy (1987) has referred to apprenticeship nurse
training as a "pipeline", which produced a group of people who had
been so thoroughly absorbed by the system that they emerged as
similar and interchangeable.

In 1994 University College Galway established the first university-
based pre-registration education programme in nursing. By 1998, all
pre-registration education of nurses in Ireland will be college-based.
The transition from the old training to the new education model has
not been trouble-free. Two particular concerns that emerged were the
methods of student selection and the front-loading of the new cur-
riculum. The University of Southampton has been commissioned by
the Department of Health and Children to evaluate the new programme in Galway. This evaluation, together with the recommendations that the Commission on Nursing will make, should ensure that
in the 21st century the career of nursing will be integrated in third-
level institutions accessed through the Central Applications Bureau.

It is imperative that a considerable proportion of nurse teaching continues to take place in clinical settings in hospitals and community. Nurse teachers will be challenged personally by the move to a college-based system and professionally by the need to ensure the integration of theory and practice in the education of nursing students. To help in bridging the theory/practice divide, teachers of nursing will need a practice base. A model on which to build might be that of the midwife teachers, some of whom continue as practitioners and hold their own clinics.

RETENTION

One factor that may hold back developments in nursing is the profession-wide response to changes in practice. In the 21st century, there will be nurses who are also behaviour therapists, community team leaders, nurse ethicists, university lecturers, nurses in care of the elderly, specialist and consultant nurses, nurse practitioners and nurses working as surgeons' assistants. This diversity of roles can only be compatible with a heterogeneous occupational group. Different nursing roles may have the same intrinsic value, but they may not be recognised and rewarded equally. However, it is possible that some nurses and unions may resist this diversification, trying to maintain the homogeneity of the nursing workforce of the 1950s, where any one nurse was interchangeable with another.

Another factor that needs acknowledgement is the difficulty in financially rewarding the nursing workforce, because their number is so large. Paying nurses, taking a homogeneous "all are equal" approach, may leave little or no room to reward nurses who have taken on additional responsibilities. Sadly, it may be the brightest and best who will be lured into higher paid jobs outside the health services. In the booming "Celtic Tiger" economy of the late 1990s, nurse managers are beginning to report increasing wastage of registered nurses. Companies who have recognised the considerable skill and talent of nurses include public relations and pharmaceutical companies. In addition, we have seen the emergence of the entrepreneur nurse who sets up and manages her own business, sometimes but not exclusively in the health area. Urgent action will have to be taken to structure salary scales to take account of nursing responsibility and specialisation.

In a market which makes recruitment and retention increasingly difficult, nurse managers will need to use the available nurses creatively, be open to the increased use of flexible hours of work, set up nursing banks within health agencies and be prepared to attract older nurses back into the nursing workforce. We may take some comfort from having approximately 20,000 additional trained nurses on the Register, at least some of whom might be persuaded to return to practice.

In *The Empty Raincoat*, Charles Handy suggests that health professionals may be drawn into a portfolio world, moving away from the valued security of the past towards the autonomy and independence of newly emerging "servant business". We are beginning to see signs of nurse entrepreneurship in Ireland. In Dublin, some younger nurses who opt to stay in nursing now prefer independence, selling their skills through a nursing agency. This gives them the freedom to decide where they will work and when. The buyers' market of the 1970s and 1980s is rapidly changing to one where nurses selling their services can pick and choose. Shortages of nurses in Europe, the United States and the Middle East have resulted in Irish nurses being in a stronger position to negotiate short contracts of employment, sometimes as short as three months.

Within Europe, Ireland leads the health litigation stakes. Our health institutions are under constant pressure to contain expenditure. Client expectation and demand continue to grow. It cannot be mere coincidence that in this climate hospitals are experiencing acute nursing shortages. Irish hospitals in the 21st century will look back with longing to the days of the institutional patriots, to a time when they had 20 applicants for every available place.

In the 20th century, cutbacks in levels of health services resulted from budgetary constraints. In the future, constraints are as likely to be the result of the institutions' inability to recruit and retain nurses with the appropriate knowledge and skill.

CONTINUING PROFESSIONAL EDUCATION

An Bord Altranais has defined continuing professional education as follows:

> Continuing education is a life long professional development process which takes place after the completion of the pre-registration nurse education programme. It consists of planned learning experiences which are designed to augment the knowledge, skills and attitude of registered nurses for the enhancement of nursing practice, patient/client care, education, administration and research (*Continuing Professional Education: A Framework*, An Bord Altranais, 1997).

Submissions by nurses to the Commission on Nursing quoted in the Interim Report refer to a lack of educational opportunities and problems with study leave. Nurses claimed that

> study leave and the payment of course fees were provided on an ad hoc basis with little consistency or equity both between organisations and within organisations (Commission on Nursing Interim Report, 1997).

Another issue that arose at the consultation meetings that the Commission held throughout the country was the lack of recognition for additional qualifications.

The demand by health agencies for specialist nurses and nurses' own awareness of the value of degree-level study indicate the importance of appropriately structured and funded opportunities for ongoing education. The Department of Health and Children recognised this in 1995. Letters of allocation for health boards and voluntary hospitals now include a specific allocation dedicated to continuing nursing education. The targeting of these monies met with varying degrees of success. This should properly be the responsibility of nurse managers. A combination of top-down and bottom-up strategies to cover both institutional-wide objectives and developmental needs of individuals would appear to be the best approach.

SPECIALISATION AND ADVANCED PRACTICE

Nurses make significant contributions to health care as a whole if they are willing to push out the boundaries of their role to meet evolving health care needs. Unfortunately, nursing has traditionally tended to be territorial. The decreasing length of hospital stay, brought about both by increasing costs and new treatment modalities, will require changes in the way nursing care is organised and delivered. Most nurses and midwives will have the opportunity to further extend their role. They have already extended their skills in areas such as phlebotomy and cannulation, suturing, ultrasonography, family planning (including the taking of smears) and in various forms of counselling and therapy. The extension of the nurse's role is to some extent the first step in a process which includes nursing specialisation and advanced nursing practice.

Currently, nurses working as specialists in all areas will usually have undertaken post-registration education. They have their own caseload of patients and may cross hospital and community boundaries. Generally, they are not part of the rostered staff in one ward or department. They provide advice and education to patients, relatives and staff. They are usually expected to undertake audit and carry out research into the services they provide.

Common areas of clinical nurse specialists in Ireland include:

- Day care cancer services
- Palliative care
- Day surgery pre-assessment clinics
- Respiratory nursing
- Stoma care
- Breast care
- Diabetic nursing
- Continence
- Lactation consultancy.

Titles can be confusing and are frequently misused. The term nurse practitioner is particularly confusing, especially to patients. Ireland has lagged behind the United States and the United Kingdom in the development of advanced nurse practitioners. Advanced nurse practitioners are registered nurses who autonomously carry out assessment and give direct primary and/or acute medical care to patients in a variety of settings. Expanding the role of nurse practitioners is a topic of great interest within the US health care industry. Many British universities now offer educational programmes for nurse practitioners, usually at Masters level. Common areas of practice for nurse practitioners include accident and emergency departments and neonatal units.

The development of nurse practitioners must be viewed as specialism as opposed to elitism. The Commission on Nursing Interim Report (1997) highlighted the fear that many nurses have about specialisation in nursing:

> It should be noted that caution was expressed during the consultative process in relation to the term "Advanced Practitioner". It was suggested that this may result in the development of a certain elitism amongst a category of nurses and more importantly may by degrees result in other nurses providing general nursing care to become seen as "basic nurses".

This apparently reactive response to a new development in nursing which has the potential to transform the profession is unfortunate, but nevertheless understandable. Nurse practitioners working within acute hospitals will considerably enhance the service provided by those hospitals. In accident and emergency departments in particular, the skills of the nurse practitioner will have considerable benefit for continuity of patient care, and reducing waiting times, which cause patients and families great distress.

The Interim Report from the Commission on Nursing did point out that developments in advanced practice "should not be seen as adding hierarchical layers but rather as a resource and opportunity for all nurses and a benefit".

MANAGEMENT IN NURSING

The group of nurses probably facing the greatest challenges in the 21st century will be nurse managers. They will be involved in recruitment, responsible for retention, lead developments in nursing and work in partnership with lecturers and teachers to ensure that nurses coming through the academic process are equipped with appropriate competencies. Among the areas requiring urgent attention from nurse managers is skill mix. In a time of increasing health service costs and difficulties with recruitment and retention, it is likely that health agencies and in particular their nurse managers will have to be creative, not just in planning services and ensuring the highest possible standards, but also in ensuring a suitable mix of skills in each specific area of practice.

In the 21st century, health service management is going to be of concern to all who work within the service. In the past, nursing management in particular tended to be narrowly focused, with progression confined to a vertical hierarchy. Flatter management structures, together with the opportunities offered by the Office for Health Management, should see nurse managers in the 21st century exploring lateral as well as vertical opportunities.

Unfortunately, Irish nurses appear to hold very negative views about their nurse managers:

> Senior nursing managements focused on such issues as rostering of nurses, sick leave and annual leave rather than on the development of nursing practice and policies for the more effective delivery of nursing care to patients. Nursing managers were preoccupied with hierarchies and the detailed control of nurses rather than the management of the function of nursing (Commission on Nursing Interim Report, 1997).

The general view of Irish nurses — that their nurse managers are disempowered — was mirrored in the opinions expressed by the nurse managers themselves. They stated that "they were under constant pressure to stay within budget". They argued that they had no involvement in setting the nursing budget and were often told that they had exceeded a budget of which they were unaware. There appeared to be a sense of "helplessness among some nurse managers because they considered that they were unable to influence corporate decision-making" (Commission on Nursing, 1997).

The establishment of the Office for Health Management in 1997 provides us with some optimism for the challenges facing nurse managers in the 21st century. In particular, the provision of master classes for senior nurse managers on "Effective Nurse Leadership: Making a Difference" is to be welcomed. Another positive initiative is the Leadership Development Programme which aims to identify and encourage young nurses (under 35) who have the potential to be future nursing leaders.

Nurses must be involved in policy-making at all levels. The first Chief Nurse was appointed to the Department of Health and Children in 1998 and hopefully will soon be followed by the appointment of nurses to the executive management structure of health boards. Nurses will also take their place on policy-making committees in hospitals and community. They will participate in clinical units of management and at ward level be facilitated to become full managers with staff and budgetary control.

COMMUNITY NURSING

The challenges facing nurses working in the community at the end of the 20th century result from the increasing cost of hospitalisation and the shift in focus from sickness to health, in current and projected national health services. Public health nurses and their managers are ideally placed to spearhead the response to these challenges. However, they must prove to policy-makers that they have the necessary expertise to plan and co-ordinate the changes that must happen, to meet new challenges. If they are not in the vanguard of proactive planning for these changes, they will be consigned to having to adapt to changes foisted upon them by others. Recognition of nurses' pivotal position in the community health services has long been articulated (Kevany, 1992). The 21st century will present public health nurses with an opportunity to demonstrate their value in the planning and managing of future service needs.

At the management level, public health nurse managers will have responsibility for the monitoring of epidemiological trends within their catchment areas. They will lead health promotion initiatives in workplace and school settings. The managers of community nursing in the 21st century will have collaborative relationships with other community leaders and work with them to effect attitudinal change towards healthier lifestyle choices.

As leaders of nursing teams, the community nurse co-ordinates and supervises different categories of carers, from home helps and home care attendants to specialist palliative care nurses working with terminally ill patients and their families. Community nurses are best placed to co-ordinate and lead the community care team. The full potential of the public health nurse's key role as co-ordinator of the various community care services should ensure that a seamless and more efficient service is given. Specialist public health nurses already exist in some areas, such as continence, breast-feeding, leg ulcer care and palliative care.

In the past, community nurses saw their role as encompassing all aspects of need within a family setting. The 21st century may see greatly expanded sub-specialisation in community nursing.

CONCLUSION

A transformation process which is already evident in Irish nursing will continue through to the 21st century. At governmental level, the issues of concern will include recruitment and retention of nurses. Methods will need to be found to remunerate nurses who take on specialist roles which must be clearly defined and adequately re-sourced. Strategies will need to be developed to minimise wastage among registered nurses.

An Bord Altranais in the 20th century tended to focus on their "gatekeeping" function, concerned with determining who could en-ter the profession and disciplining those who fail to meet standards. In the 21st century, it will be concerned with preventing poor prac-tice and supporting good practice, which should in turn reduce the focus on discipline. How to regulate speciality and advanced practice properly will need to be addressed. In an environment of rapid changes in technology, continuing competence will be of critical importance and is likely to require mandatory continuing education. The Board will need to establish standards for practice, which set out minimum expectations, in order to fulfil its function to protect the public. This will facilitate the Board in upholding the integrity of the profession and will support nursing's contribution to society.

Nurse managers in the 21st century will be concerned with management and practice issues including:

- Specialisation in practice;

- A shift from institutional to primary care;

- Ensuring continuing competence in all practice settings in an environment of rapidly advancing technology;

- Ensuring that non-professional care providers are adequately educated and supervised and given only appropriate responsibilities.

Nurse managers must develop new leadership approaches, such as shared governance, appropriate to the management of a professional occupational group.

In late-20th-century Ireland, nurses have been concerned with such issues as rotas, permanency, pay, promotional opportunities and defending the existence of a nursing hierarchy. In the 21st century, they are more likely to seek job enhancement; autonomy; empowerment; recognition of their complementary rather than subsidiary relationship with medicine; remuneration for added responsibility and specialisation; and to have the opportunity to participate in shared governance of their hospital or community care area.

In the 20th century the first person a patient met in the accident and emergency department of an acute hospital was most likely a nurse, whose task it was to explain and excuse why they might have to wait several hours because the doctors were busy. In 21st century Ireland, this nurse will be able to carry out preliminary investigation and treatment for many patients, complementing and supporting the work of doctors and providing a more timely, seamless and acceptable service.

References

An Bord Altranais (1997), *Continuing Professional Education: A Framework*, Dublin: An Bord Altranais.

Commission on Nursing Interim Report (1997), Dublin: Government Publications Office.

Dwyer, M. (1983), "Nursing in Ireland", *Nursing Mirror*, Vol. 156, p. 21.

Handy, C. (1994), *The Empty Raincoat: Making Sense of the Future*, London: Hutchinson.

Kevany, J. (1992), "Who is Responsible for Care in the Community?" Proceedings of the Conference on the Future of Community Health Nursing, Limerick: Mid-Western Health Board.

McCarthy, G. (1988), "Student Nurses in the Republic of Ireland: A Study of their Biographical, Educational, Motivational and Personality Characteristics, Unpublished M.Ed. dissertation, Trinity College Dublin.

Nursing Applications Centre (1997), "Review of Operations", Dublin: Price Waterhouse.

OECD (1997), *Economic Surveys — Ireland 1996–1997*, Paris: OECD.

Styles, M.M. (1997), "International Differences in Politics, Healthcare and Regulation", Proceedings of the Third International Conference on the Regulation of Nursing and Midwifery, Geneva: International Council of Nurses.

Treacy, M.M. (1987), "In the Pipeline: A Qualitative Study of General Nurse Training with Special Reference to Nurses' Role in Health Education" Unpublished PhD Dissertation, University of London Institute of Education.

PART FOUR

Leadership

15

FORM FOLLOWS FUNCTION: ADAPTING HEALTH MANAGEMENT STRUCTURES TO ACHIEVE HEALTH AND SOCIAL GAINS

Denis Doherty

INTRODUCTION

The debate about how the health services in Ireland should be structured and managed went on for years. Did we really need eight health boards? Should the programme system be replaced by a system of geographical management? Given the amount of money we were spending on health care, why was the citizen not receiving a more comprehensive service? These were all valid questions; the problem was that the key question was not posed.

Good evidence existed that "form should follow function" but we did not seriously consider what function our health services should perform. There was broad agreement that there should be a shift from hospital care towards community care and that we should be doing more to promote good health. Spending on community-based services and health promotion had indeed increased, in real terms, but, in relative terms, hospital services retained their dominant position.

The long-awaited health strategy was to prove a remarkably enlightened and farsighted document. Published in 1994, *Shaping a Healthier Future* placed the emphasis on health rather than on health services and adopted the concepts of health gain and social gain to describe what the function of the health services should be. The principles of equity, quality and accountability underpin the Strategy. *Thus, the health services should be structured so as to maximise the achievement of health and social gain.* This chapter considers the principles which should guide the development of health management structures to the next century.

INVESTING FOR SOCIAL RETURN

At the time the Strategy was published, there was a trend towards privatisation of some public services in Ireland. Services which were to remain publicly funded were expected to be able to demonstrate standards of efficiency and effectiveness comparable to their counterparts in the commercial sector. Comparisons between commercial organisations and the health services are difficult to make but are made somewhat easier as a result of adopting the concepts of health gain and social gain. Commercial concerns exist to produce a financial return on the investments of their shareholders and the role of management is to produce financial results. Citizens, as taxpayers, are the investors in the health services. They are promised a social return on their investment in the form of improvements in the health status of the population They are offered dividends in the form of entitlements to services when they need them. The role of health services management in that context is to produce social results in the form of health gains and social gains.

There remains the difficulty that, while financial returns and results are easy to measure and understand, social results are not. The concept of health gain is valuable in that regard too. Continued investment or new investment can only be justified if it can be shown to contribute an acceptable level of health or social gain. The importance of being able to demonstrate the evidence base in policy, management and clinical decision-making is becoming more accepted. Instruments and techniques are being devised which are improving our ability to assemble and demonstrate the evidence. In another field, the Environmental Impact Study has been devised to calculate the impact a proposed development will have on the environment, thereby demonstrating that measurements previously considered too difficult to undertake can be made. Can we avoid developing a similar technique — the health gain impact study — to guide investment in health care? After all, a high proportion of our national wealth is already spent on health care and the capacity of health care systems to consume resources appears insatiable.

The health strategy acknowledges that health gain is not achievable by the health services alone. The major causes for morbidity and mortality in Ireland are largely related to lifestyles. The health services are well placed to identify and quantify the causes of ill health and to contribute, by way of providing advice, to approaches aimed at promoting better health. However, Ireland is a free country and citizens, policy-makers and legislators can choose to ignore advice, even when the available evidence is overwhelming. For example, smoking is a major cause of serious illness, death and expense on our health services, but we lag behind other countries in our attempts to discourage smoking. Many non-smokers are remarkably tolerant of passive smoking, even in designated non-smoking areas. On the other hand, citizens sometimes become very concerned about issues which are of low risk to their health. The citizen, like the customer, is entitled to be accepted as being always right. *The health gain challenge is to devise means and structures to promote cross-sectoral/interorganisational alliances devoted to reducing risks to health.*

When we speak of health and social gains we are, realistically, limited to relative improvements, at least in the short term. Given that our health prospects are determined at a young age, or even before we are born in some respects, health improvements may have to be measured in terms of the extent to which interventions moderate the progress of illness or disability. One of the many paradoxes we face in health care is that, as general economic standards improve, the incidence of poverty-induced illnesses reduces and the incidence of affluence-related illnesses increases. Another is that, as more patients survive previously fatal illnesses, thanks to improvements in medical knowledge and hospital practices, the cost to the health services increases because of the costs associated with maintaining the patients' adjusted health status.

The Health Strategy, by adopting the principles of equity, quality and accountability, emphasises that ours is a state-wide health system and not just eight separate centrally funded systems. For service delivery purposes, there are eight health boards, each of which is responsible for a defined geographical area. These areas, which were formed in 1970, are familiar to the people they serve. This fact, coupled with an acknowledgement that delivery structures only facilitate performance of the tasks to be carried out, influenced the decision to retain the eight boards network. The Strategy emphasised that, in future, closer co-operation between boards would be expected. This has since become a legal obligation.

BALANCING ACCOUNTABILITY FOR SPENDING PUBLIC FUNDS AND MEETING CITIZEN ENTITLEMENTS

As they pursue health gains for the populations which they serve, health boards also have to comply with more stringent accountability standards. They have become more accountable to the system for the way they spend public money and they are becoming more accountable to the citizen in respect of the citizen's entitlements. Words such as greater openness and transparency are being used to describe the changes that are well underway. In terms of accountability for the spending of public money, health boards have come within the remit of the Comptroller and Auditor General (C&AG). In that regard, they operate accounting standards which are broadly comparable to those in the private sector. The C&AG's role includes value for money (VFM) audits. A number of VFM audits have compared how particular services are organised in each of the boards and the results being achieved. That approach is compatible with the principles of equity, quality and accountability which underpin the strategy, and boards need to bear that in mind when reviewing their structures.

The Health (Amendment) Act, 1996, imposes a statutory obligation on boards to co-operate in areas of common interest. That same legislation deals comprehensively with relationships between boards and the Department of Health and Children, and between boards and their chief executive officers. The service plan is the mechanism chosen to structure those relationships. The service plan, the audit report and the annual report, now a statutory requirement, taken together amount to the means by which the individual citizen, or the citizen's watchdog, The Public Accounts Committee, can examine a particular board's observance of its obligations to be held accountable. *The appropriateness of the structures in place will have a bearing on a board's ability to comply with its overall accountability obligations.* The Service Plan has the potential to become a mechanism by which the health care system can secure measurable health gains for the people of Ireland. However, it also has the potential to stifle progress if the approach were to become one of concern only with the narrower technical aspects of accountability. The challenge is to achieve a good balance between the need to achieve social returns on investments in health care and the requirement to be publicly accountable for the spending of the monies involved.

In addition, the desired balance should satisfy the entitlements of citizens. The Ombudsman Act, the Patients Charter and the Freedom of Information Act are examples of how the entitlements of citizens have been more explicitly provided for in recent years. Taken together, they form a comprehensive guide to citizens on the response they can expect to receive from state agencies and services of the state. Health services providers could take the view that, by providing appropriate systems, procedures or structures, they could comply with their specific obligations. A more enlightened approach will view the new legislation as developing guidance for public officials on the type of relationships the state wishes to have with its citizens in their dealings with the public services. All the indications are that future relationships between the citizen and the state and its agencies will be more open and transparent and this has implications for the way public service organisations do their business. There is an evolutionary process at work which public officials must, at worst, understand and preferably should lead. Because that evolution is set to continue, *structures need to be flexible so that the relationship between the organisation and the citizens it serves can continue to grow. These structures also need to contain elements that will guarantee the citizens the minimum that they are entitled to receive and the redress open to them should they feel aggrieved.*

FUTURE ROLES — DEPARTMENT, HEALTH BOARDS, NON-STATUTORY PROVIDERS

The role of the Department of Health and Children is set to change. In future, the Department will concern itself with policy formation, supporting the Minister and evaluating the effectiveness of our health services. The health boards' remit will be extended to include the range of functions currently carried out by the Department which do not come within its new role. Many of our health services are delivered by non-statutory providers; examples include most acute care services in Dublin and services for the mentally handicapped throughout the state. There are many other examples of high quality services delivered by non-statutory providers. Traditionally, the larger of these providers were funded directly by the Department of Health. In keeping with their responsibilities for the health of the populations of their areas, the health boards will in future fund these non-statutory providers of health services in their areas. They are to be renamed health authorities to reflect this new role. The Eastern Health Board, because of the size of the population it serves and the extent to which services are delivered by non-statutory providers, is to be restructured. This work is being undertaken by a Task Force appointed by the Minister for Health. Legislation will be needed to give effect to the new arrangements.

In light of the fact that the boards will provide some services directly and that other services will be provided by non-statutory providers, funding arrangements must ensure that the non-statutory providers receive fair treatment. That involves two main considerations. One relates to acknowledging the vital contribution non-statutory organisations have made to the development of our services, as well as recognising their expertise and commitment to the work in which they are engaged and their potential to enrich the process of assuring population health. *The second involves the putting in place of structures which will ensure parity of treatment of the statutory and non-statutory providers in the allocation of resources and in monitoring the effectiveness and quality of services delivered.*

ASSESSING AND PRIORITISING NEEDS

In shifting the focus from health services to health itself, it becomes necessary to know what the health needs of the population served are and to tailor services to satisfy those needs. In health care, everywhere, resources are frequently secured on the strength of the case made by those working in specialist areas. The promising new drug therapy which may arrest the progress of a fatal illness will often attract funding easier than, say, a service for the elderly, which has to be rationed because the amount of money available to it is insufficient to meet the needs of the service. As medical knowledge and technology continue to improve, the health services are likely to be faced even more than they are now with having to make choices. Even though the word "rationing" is disliked, rationing is practiced in our health services just as it is in every other health care system. Until now, it has been largely implicit. However, as the trend towards greater openness and transparency develops, we are likely to be called upon to be more explicit where rationing is concerned. In any event, it is entirely reasonable that a health care system, which exists with a mission to improve the health of the population, should have in place arrangements to inform policy-makers which services and interventions should attract funding, based on their potential to satisfy need. *The boards will need to develop structures to enable them to meet their population health responsibilities.* This will involve both assessing what the health needs of the population are and service commissioning so that the available resources are deployed in ways which impact most on the needs which have been identified. The skills and talents of public health specialists, policy analysts, researchers, health economists, quality assurers and service providers will have to be deployed and combined in teams in the task of assuring population health. It is unlikely that boards will retain staff, full time, in all of the specialities involved; nor is it likely that the composition of teams will remain constant. The structures chosen will need to be flexible so that the appropriate mix of talents and skills can be assembled to undertake particular tasks and be dismantled when that task has been completed.

GREATER FLEXIBILITY

Flexibility will become more important in the period ahead. Population health and accountability imperatives will demand that. *Structures will have to be capable of managing the whole of the business of the boards; that is, assuring population health.* That will be accomplished by teams with a task focus. Teams are increasingly likely to be formed to perform specific tasks and be disbanded when the tasks they were set up to do have been completed. Senior managers may at any time be members of a number of teams and hold a board-wide remit for a specific aspect of a board's population health responsibilities. A management-by-programmes approach is, therefore, outdated.

That concept of a management team in health boards was introduced by the management consultants, McKinsey, in 1971 and remains in place to a greater or lesser extent to the present time. As the range and complexity of the services provided by the boards expanded, so too did the membership of the teams. This resulted in an undesireable and unintended increase in the span of control. The distinctions still in use between team members as line managers and team members as functional officers is not conducive to managing the health gain agenda. It is a measure of the flexible attitudes adopted by management team members in recent years that so much change has been smoothly accomplished.

FEDERALISM IN HEALTH CARE DELIVERY

Even the smallest of the health boards is, by any standards, a large and very complex organisation. The 1998 budget of the Midland Health Board exceeds £130 million and it employs 3,400 staff directly and a further 1,000 in services delivered by non-statutory organisations.

A single hospital, not to mention a health board, is a highly complex organisation. Management gurus Peter Drucker, Sir John Harvey Jones and Henry Mintzberg have all concluded that hospital and health care management is exceedingly difficult. When funding was less of an issue than it is today, the way hospitals were organised and managed attracted little attention. Hospitals are now being asked to demonstrate that they have changed in the way industrial and commercial organisations have in recent years, in response to public demand for greater efficiency and effectiveness.

In his book *The Empty Raincoat*, Charles Handy includes a quotation from Homa Bahrami which describes how a hospital or a health board might become:

> a federation or constellation of business units that are typically interdependent, relying on one another for critical expertise and know-how. The centre's role is to orchestrate the broad strategic vision, develop the shared administrative and organisational infrastructure, and create the cultural gene which can create synergies.

Bahrami was, in fact, describing the new high-tech companies in Silicon Valley.

That is not how health boards and hospitals in Ireland have functioned in the past. The year 1997 will be remembered as one of unrest in Irish hospitals. Serious industrial relations disputes involved nurses and paramedical staff. The consultants' contract was finally renegotiated towards the end of the year and contains provisions intended to improve the management of hospitals through the active involvement of consultants.The financial settlements arrived at cost a great deal of money. There remained, however, a wide range of unresolved issues that were referred to a Commission on Nursing and an Expert Group on paramedical staff.

Nurses in Ireland are highly thought of by members of the public. It is surprising, then, to be told by representatives of the profession that they feel undervalued and suffer from low self-esteem as a profession. There is a widely held view that the role of the profession is ill-defined and poorly understood within the health services. The profession is self-regulated, but there is widespread dissatisfaction with the regulatory body. Many believe that, because hospital consultants are still mainly male and nurses are predominately female, the changes which have resulted in greater equality between men and women in Irish society in recent decades have not been achieved in hospitals, as workplaces.

The nursing profession attracts many very bright entrants and many in the profession are committed to continuing education and personal development. They encounter frustrations in dealing with workloads which, on the one hand, require them to undertake some tasks which could be performed by less skilled staff and, on the other hand, precludes them from performing tasks that they consider themselves capable of but which must be performed by doctors.

Resolution of issues of this nature will remain difficult as long as professional boundaries, which owe more to their historical origins and custom and practice than to today's needs, remain unchanged. The "Tierney Report" (1993) on medical manpower has been debated for over two years now. However, the profession remains divided on its recommendations and it appears unclear when and how conclusions leading to action will be arrived at. The Report of the Commission on Nursing will, no doubt, deal fully with the issues of concern to the nursing profession. The key question of how best to meet the needs of patients in future may not be adequately addressed until the roles of the many professions who contribute to patient care are considered together. The Irish doctor, like the Irish nurse, the Irish physiotherapist and other health care professionals, is rightly highly regarded at home and abroad. The maintenance of these high professional reputations into the future may depend on the willingness of the professions themselves to recognise the advantages to be gained from structured inter-professional co-operation predicated on a commitment to optimising patient care.

As Irish people, we are comfortable in federal arrangements. Our native townland, parish and county are important to most of us and we often go to great lengths to sustain our links with them. As members of the European Union, we are committed Europeans, but in a way which also emphasises our Irishness. We are intensely proud of the "Celtic Tiger" economy at home and of the reputation for hard work enjoyed by Irish people abroad. Federation is an ancient concept which is remarkably relevant to the challenges and opportunities the health services face. *It would be remarkably shortsighted not to consider the potential contribution of federalism in devising structures at local, area and national levels in the pursuit of health gain.*

Box 15.1: Federal Arrangements Involving Nurses, as an Example

It is not unusual or surprising that members of staff find it easier to identify with the unit they work in than with the board that employs them. It is laudable that, for example, a nurse working in a residential centre for the elderly should identify almost totally with that unit. After all, the unit exists to care for the elderly patients there, whose needs are best met in that residential care setting. The unit is, of course, also part of a network of services the health board provides to meet the care needs of older people. It is important, therefore, that staff of the unit understand how their unit fits into the overall scheme of things and how the work they do individually serves not only the patients they care for directly but also the larger group of older people who benefit from residential care. As part of what is a national health service, their unit is part of Irish society's contribution to the care of older people. That adds up to a federation of interests. The nurse, in this example, devotes her professional skills to the patients of the local unit. She is employed by the health board as part of the board's pursuit of health gain and social gain for older people and she is also part of the national health service for older people. The principles on which that service is founded are, firstly, that older people in the geographical area served by the unit should have access to services they need comparable to those available to their counterparts in other areas; and, secondly, that the quality of the care should also be comparable with that provided by other units. Of course, as a nurse, she is also a member of the largest and one of the most important professions involved in health care. Her interests, therefore, extend to a variety of other health care areas where nurses are employed and include the role and development of her profession. She therefore finds herself in a number of federal arrangements, as do many other professionals working in our health services.

CHANGING CUSTOM AND PRACTICE

A number of Irish hospitals are piloting new organisational arrangements using directorates of services. In other health care systems, where directorates have existed for some time, they are considered by many to have improved the service patients receive and have contributed to closer and more meaningful interprofessional working. While respecting the clinical autonomy of the doctor, they allow the roles of the other professionals to evolve through closer working, better communication and greater local autonomy. That greater autonomy stems from the authority which the directorate has as a business unit that has vested in it a well-developed role and authority to make decisions within overall hospital policies and accountability requirements. *That structure is an example of form following function, but it need not become universally adopted as being the only or best structure.* Social entrepreneurship ought to be encouraged in the health and social services. *If the staff of a hospital agree an approach and structures that they believe will best serve the patients of their hospital, their proposals should be assessed and facilitated if they are accepted as having merit.* The likely impact on staff commitment ought to be weighed against the accepted orthodoxy of structures when experimentation is mooted.

Box 15.2: A Form of Social Entrepreneurship

Let us take the management of waiting lists to illustrate how established practice can be overwhelmed when demand exceeds supply and how solutions can benefit from problem-solving approaches and new alliances. Hospitals tend to have an established approach to the way they do things. Administrative custom and practice and professional relationships tend to be important. Such ways of doing things tend to work well when there is balance between supply and demand. They tend to be inflexible when problems arise. Waiting lists have become a cause of concern in a number of specialities and have given rise to a great deal of public debate. They have been on the national political agenda for some years and have attracted additional earmarked funding.

The established practice which is involved here is that general practitioners refer patients to hospitals when they require a consultant's opinion. This arrangement works best when the volume of referrals from general practitioners matches the capacity of the consultant service to see new referrals. Smallish waiting lists are not a problem, since they do not use much of the consultants' time for their management. As lists grow, the problem increases and becomes more complex when service standards aim at, for example, adults not having to wait more than twelve months and children not more than six months. A problem general practitioners face is that there is no mechanism to inform them of either waiting lists size or waiting times. They are not, as a rule, involved in the management of waiting lists or in prioritising the relative urgency of patients referred from their practices. Where long waiting lists exist, it seems more sensible that the consultants be facilitated to devote the bulk of their working time to dealing with their clinical work than in having to spend an inordinate amount of time in managing the lists. The answer is not to assign this important task to medical secretaries whose talents lie in the area of administration. Those who know the patients best, the referring general practitioners, are not, as a rule, afforded any role in prioritising which patients should be attended to soonest. Until such time as waiting lists have been disposed of, the emphasis must be on using the available resources to deal with those patients whose needs are greatest. That requires a willingness to put structures in place capable of dealing with the task in hand, even if that involves changing custom and practice.

Professor Henry Mintzberg, writing in the Fall 1997 issue of *Health Care Management Review*, said:

> hospitals are constantly reorganising, which means shuffling boxes around on pieces of paper. Somehow it is believed that by rearranging authority relationships, problems will be solved. But all this may reflect no more than the frustration of managers in trying to effect real change in the clinical operations. Architecture might offer a much more effective solution. If even a fraction of the efforts that are put into moving positions around on charts went into moving people around on floors, there might be a lot more collaborative activities in hospitals.

MANAGING KNOWLEDGE

Today, some hospitals are described as being high-tech and, therefore, considered to be well endowed with the latest equipment and the technicians needed to operate them. It is much less usual to hear hospitals referred to as "high knowledge" institutions and little attention is paid to how the knowledge an institution possesses should be managed. Data management is, in practice, restricted to the management of information and it is rare to view knowledge as an asset worthy of being qualified, valued and exploited in the way other resources are. Knowledge, as a corporate asset, has the potential to contribute much to the attainment of social results in the future. Just how much potential it offers is difficult to predict and, therefore, merits being viewed as a subject worthy of study and investment appraisal in its own right.

INFLUENCE OF EUROPEAN UNION

Our membership of the European Union has not, until now, been a consideration in our discussion on either health or health care issues. The interpretation of the concept of subsidiarity has resulted in acceptance that health care is the responsibility of the individual member states. At the same time, public health is seen more and more as an issue which should be addressed by the EU as a whole. Prior to the Maastricht Treaty, the European Commission was seen as having only very limited competency in the field of health care. In the intervening period, the competency of the Commission has grown and is set to expand further when the Treaty of Amsterdam is ratified. It is difficult to predict how far these changes will extend, but it seems reasonable to assume that citizens of the European Union in one member state will expect to be eligible for health care benefits comparable with the best available in other member states. Will not citizens on waiting lists for treatment demand to be allowed to avail of services in another member state where it is not necessary to wait for treatment? As an island community, we may not be among the first to have to address these issues, but nonetheless we need to maintain a watching brief on developments so that our citizens are afforded opportunities to avail of the health care benefits to be derived from our membership of the European Union.

IMPORTANCE OF ACHIEVING BALANCE

For the foreseeable future, however, our health services will continue to be financed by our government and will be refocused to improve the health status of the Irish people by using the available resources in ways that produce the best results. It is a national health system founded on the principles of equity, quality and accountability. Nevertheless, service delivery is to be decentralised. The Department of Health and Children will concern itself mainly with policy formation, legislation, supporting the Minister and monitoring service quality. The health boards will have overall responsibility for meeting the health needs of the populations they serve. They will provide some services directly and others by arrangement with non-statutory providers. In the case of the services that they will provide directly, they will have to determine the degree of autonomy they will afford the individual service units. The health boards will be required to work conjointly in pursuit of population health targets to a very much greater extent than they have in the past.

Almost certainly, federalism, even if it is not specifically acknowledged, is likely to feature strongly in shaping future arrangements and at many levels; for example,

- The Department of Health and Children and individual health boards;

- The Department and all of the health boards;

- A health board and non-statutory providers of services for people with disabilities;

- A health board and its acute hospitals;

- Departments or directorates of hospitals with each other.

The desired balance, in whatever new relationships are formed, will have to be carefully developed and supported. The Department of Health and Children, the health boards and the larger acute hospitals will all have to address similar key questions, such as: how much can be devolved and how the centre can provide the organisational glue which ensures that the whole of what is achieved is greater than the sum of the individual parts. The units to which functions will be devolved will in turn need to recognise the value of a strong, though small centre. Again, Charles Handy deals with the paradox involved in his book *The Empty Raincoat*:

> In a business it may make good logical sense to combine functions, to group some regions together, to manage cash or purchasing centrally, but these actions all steal power from the independent units. Those units will resent this, not understanding the paradox that, in order to get the most value out of their independence, it often pays to sacrifice some of that independence to a central function. That kind of compromise is only done willingly if there is some confidence in the central function, some sense of belonging to a larger whole of which it, too, is part.

That larger whole, in the case of health services, is population health. A claim to independence is not sustainable unless it is in the interest of achieving measurable health gain.

The importance of teamworking, as a means of achieving results in health care, has been recognised for many years. In practice, the results attributable to teamworking have been disappointing. When a team is formed, it ought to be for a clearly stated purpose. Members of the team ought to be clear about the roles they are expected to perform. It is unreasonable to expect talented individuals to perform well as a team. Strong leadership and skilled coaching are invariably ingredients in the success of winning teams, in sport, in business and in entertainment. In the past, the ex officio authority that a manager's place in the hierachy bestowed was often confused with leadership. Respect and credibility has to be earned and leaders need to be developed and nutured. In the past, investment in training has not been matched by investment in coaching. *The achievement of measurable outcomes — health and social gains — in more flexibly structured organisations will benefit from good coaching.*

The Management Development Strategy, published in 1997, saw the need to strengthen management capacity, in the health services, as crucial to achieving improvements in the health of the population. The Minister for Health and Children immediately established the Office for Health Management. The Office has prioritised the development of leaders and managers and expanding opportunities for women in management for early attention. In recognition of the fact that the health profession attracts many of the most able and talented school leavers and that, based on experience to date, many of the senior managers of the future will emerge from within the system, strong emphasis is being placed on identifying, coaching and developing young leaders.

CONCLUSION

The overall mission is very clear and the ways of going about fulfilling the mission are becoming clearer. There is now an emphasis on care groups rather than on programmes of services, for example. *Teams, not individuals, will become the building blocks of organisations pursuing health gains.* The teams will be assembled by drawing together the skills and experience needed to undertake a particular task. The policy statement will need to be converted to operational programmes and responsibilities for implementation specifically assigned. *Structures need to be viewed as merely the framework or scaffolding for allowing the work of the organisation to get done.* Builders erect a structure of steel scaffolding to facilitate the work of putting in place the permanent structure for which they have contracted. When the permanent structure is in place, they dismantle the scaffolding and move it to another building site. Over the years, scaffolding has become lighter, more flexible and affords more protection to construction workers. *Structures in hospitals and health services need to become more flexible and afford more protection also.* They need to be designed and assembled to perform a particular task, and dismantled when the task has been completed. They should be dismantled and replaced if they are not affording the level of protection which they were designed to provide. Scaffolding on a building site is determined by the architectural drawings for the project. In other words, form follows function. *In the health services, the need for form to follow function should be the primary consideration in devising structures.* That will remain as valid in the next millennium as it has in this. Leadership and coaching skills will replace the ex officio authority which the manager's place in the hierachy once bestowed.

References

An Oireachtas, *Comptroller and Auditor General (Amendment) Act, 1993*, Dublin: Government Publications.

An Oireachtas, *Freedom of Information Act, 1997*, Dublin: Government Publications.

An Oireachtas, *Ombudsman Act, 1980*, Dublin: Government Publications.

An Oireachtas, *Health Amendment (No. 3) Act, 1996*, Dublin: Government Publications.

Beckhard, Richard, and Wendy Pritchard (1992), *Changing the Essence. The Art of Creating and Leading Fundamental Change in Organisations*, San Francisco: Jossey-Bass Publishers.

Department of Health (1994), *Shaping a Healthier Future. A Strategy for Effective Healthcare in the 1990s*, Dublin: Stationery Office.

Dixon, Dr Maureen and Dr Alison Baker, Healthcare Risk Solutions Ltd. (1996), *A Management Development Strategy for the Health and Personal Social Services in Ireland*, Dublin: Department of Health.

Drucker, Peter F. (1992), "The New Society of Organisations", *Harvard Business Review*, September–October.

Handy, Charles (1994), *The Empty Raincoat: Making Sense of the Future*, London: Hutchinson.

Marmor, Theodore R. (1997), "Changing Conditions for Healthcare Management, or Hope and Hyperbole: The Rhetoric and Reality of Managerial Reform in Health Care", European Healthcare Management Assoc. Conference.

Mintzberg, Henry (1997), "Toward Healthier Hospitals", *Healthcare Management Review*, Vol. 22, No. 40, pp. 9–18.

Tierney Report (Department of Health, Comhairle na nOspidéal and Postgraduate Medical and Dental Board) (1993), "Medical Manpower in Acute Hospitals: a Discussion Document", June.

16

INTEGRATING DOCTORS AND MANAGERS

David McCutcheon

INTRODUCTION

While doctors have always been advocates of greater quality of care and administrators have been concerned with the allocation and marshalling of resources, they share a common desire to provide high quality care. The unifying force for involvement of doctors in management is in the realisation that involvement will bring about improved outcomes for patients. The issues of equity and accountability will be resolved on the coat tails of resolving quality issues.

Although quality of care is the common motivation for involvement in health system development, the administrator and the doctor have, however, approached quality from opposite poles in the past. The doctor wished to see the results of the caring process while the administrator maintained a focus on the resources consumed in the caring process. For a considerable amount of time, they were both content in a separate existence. A profound change of role will develop in the next century for the administrator and the doctor, yielding a unification within the process of care.

There is now a realisation that the doctor and the administrator have needs that must be reconciled. The needs for the doctor are to provide high quality care in an environment that permits freedom to make clinical decisions, is conducive to the realisation of professional goals, recognises specialisation and provides accountability and peer review. The needs for the administrator are planning and control of cost, use of resources through defined authority structures and empowerment through communication improvement and participation in decision-making. Doctors are increasingly being drawn to an involvement in management.

The big challenge for doctors is to enter management realising that they must shed the coat of the doctor, representing the doctor's mindset, and take on a new cloak. The doctor arriving into management brings a scientific mind to the management process. However, the practice of management has a greater mix of art than science, which can prove quite discomforting for doctors.

Doctors and managers historically had a fundamental lack of understanding of each other. They approached each other with different experiences: the doctor in science, the manager in practice. They also had different perspectives: the doctor on outcomes, the manager on structure and process. This considerable gap must be bridged through an improved understanding of the contribution that each can make to quality patient care. The doctor's contribution is through an understanding of the clinical impact of decisions. The manager's lot is in financial planning and organisational understanding.

Doctors approach management in several ways. They may sit on the boards of organisations. They may contribute through committee structures and through strategic management decisions. Finally, doctors can be involved in day-to-day operations of health care agencies. The input, therefore, can be on the basis of policy, strategic management or operations.

The most important challenge is to discover a mechanism by which the respective interests of management and doctors can meet. This meeting of minds can occur in the spectrum of quality management. Quality management is the most fundamental focus of any health care organisation and provides the vehicle for the participation in management of both administrators and doctors, resulting in the needs of patients being served. The changing emphasis from providers to patients will also help focus doctors and administrators. Quality management incorporates eight dimensions and in order to improve the quality of care, these need to be measured and managed. The administrator and doctor will have different perspectives on each of the eight dimensions of quality, yet if each has a common understanding of a quality model, a unified approach is possible.

MANAGING SAFETY

Every patient coming to hospital or into any care process expects the care process to be safe. Why would patients subject themselves to anaesthesia unless the procedure was deemed to be safe? They expect that every risk is managed in a way that only the patient's own biological risks prevail.

Managing risks can be done by simply paying insurance, but more and more insurers are specifying risk reduction activities in order to reduce premiums. Clinical risk management is an area that brings the administrator and the doctor together.

Risk management involves equipment safety, environmental and occupational health and safety. The merger of administrative and clinical activities occurs in infection control and in critical incident debriefing and review. Some institutions still practise under separate clinical and other risk programmes, while the most progressive have migrated into an integrated "loss prevention" programme. The latter requires a comprehensive integrated risk programme, with administrative and clinical issues managed in an interdisciplinary way.

MANAGING COMPETENCE

This is one area where there will soon be a revolution in Irish medicine. The rate of generation of new information and the rate of change in technology is rapid. The changing clinical role of professions is profound. How do clinical managers cope with these types of changes? Given the emphasis on accountability in the health strategy and the harsh litigation environment, how will we provide the Minister of Health with the system of accountability that our community will demand in the next century?

The answers lie in having systems in place which ensure that professional competence is maintained. Competence has three dimensions: knowledge, skill and aptitude, which includes attitude. The new role for doctors will include development of programmes to recruit competent professionals, which will require an effective recruitment process and an equally effective process to ensure competence is maintained.

Loss of competence can occur through diseases such as alcoholism or dementing illness. It can also occur through atrophy of skill or a failure to retain knowledge. Carefully managed performance appraisal systems will evolve out of a peer review system. The role of managing competence will require great leadership and a supportive environment.

MANAGING ACCEPTABILITY

Doctors are perceived to be professional in their approach to providing care and ensuring that it is incorporated into the philosophy of education in medicine. The manager looks at quality of service in terms of how the patient, customer or client perceives care provision and seeks to optimise the acceptability of the care delivery system. It can be extremely difficult for doctors to reconcile the meeting of the demands of the profession with the acceptability of the care delivery to the patient.

These are different perspectives on the same issue. Patients' perceptions of their needs can contrast quite significantly with the doctor's perception of patients' needs. The manager and the doctor can consequently differ over the whole concept of managing the acceptability of care. The patient undergoing anaesthesia assumes that both the surgeon and the anaesthetist are completely competent to deliver the care; however, they assess that competence through the personal contact of the surgeons and the anaesthetists. The patient expects the service to be provided in an acceptable way.

Managing acceptability is a significant stretch for care providers. They have traditionally relied on verbal feedback from patients and families. A meeting of minds has to take place with regard to systems of feedback from patients and families and eventually in a formal review process of acceptability of care.

ACCESSIBILITY TO CARE

Managing accessibility to care is a significant area of concern for both the manager and the doctor. The doctor may contend that a waiting list is a pure indicator of a lack of resources. The administrator, coming to it from the perspective of resource conservation, will look at the efficiency in which the patients can enter and exit care delivery systems. The use of queuing theory (a tool and technique of management science) can indeed assist the administrator and doctor to provide care more efficiently and effectively.

In the past, administrators have focused on the length of stay of patients. The doctor's perspective saw the issue in terms of length of time from initial presentation of an illness, to diagnosis, to treatment and discharge from care. The concept of the continuum of care was not previously in the administrator's domain, as they took responsibility for their own area, e.g. primary, secondary or tertiary care. The health system in the next century will embrace the concept of networks, yielding another meeting of minds.

MANAGING EFFICIENCY

In economic terms, efficiency can be defined as the ratio between outputs and inputs. In translating this to health care delivery systems, efficiency is defined as the use of the least resource possible to achieve a given outcome. The quality component is that efficient use of a resource means that there is more available to provide care for others.

In the future, clinical pathways algorithms and clinical practice guidelines will be used as mechanisms through which the goals of the doctor and the administrator can meet. The doctor will understand a little about finance and a lot about the finite availability of resources. The administrator will understand a little more about the continuum of care.

MANAGING APPROPRIATENESS

Managing appropriateness will bring about another challenge to all in the health system. How will we decide who gets a particular resource and who does not? As doctors, we understand that sometimes care is not appropriate, but we manage this on an individual basis. The difficulty lies in the appropriate allocation of a treatment to a group of individuals and in the ethical dimension of resources.

MANAGING EFFECTIVENESS

The management of effectiveness will bring about considerable challenges for all. The challenge for the doctor is to convince the administrator that the latest is indeed the best. The immediate response may be that the best is too expensive and the administrator may hide behind cost-benefit analysis. Rigorous assessment of new technologies will become routine in the next century. This will help to provide the necessary evidence for the development of more effective treatments.

MANAGING CONTINUITY

Continuity of care will pose the greatest difficulty for health care in the 21st century. How will we handle the transfer of patients from one place of care to another? Administrators and doctors tend to approach this aspect of quality poorly, as both tend to manage within their own area of responsibility. The solution will lie in the integration of health care systems. There will be a seamless structure providing primary, secondary, tertiary and long-term care.

The impetus for this integration will come from those who pay, i.e. governments and insurers. The important issue is that, whatever the impetus, the transfer of care will be managed well from the medical and administrative perspectives, to ensure that the patient gets the best care.

THE REQUIRED STRUCTURES

The pursuit of a quality agenda needs supporting management structures. At present, doctors and administrators tend to work in separate structures, thus clouding the accountability issue and creating difficulty in communications.

There is some empirical evidence of improving work satisfaction and enhancing patient satisfaction through integrating structures. The introduction of programme management or clinical directorates are examples of such integrating structures. These provide for leadership where decisions on quality of care, volume of service and the allocation of available resources are made by those directly involved in the care of patients.

The move to programmes or clinical directorates will require a considerable investment by all concerned. For the doctor, the investment is in education and time diverted from clinical practice. The manager needs to introduce considerable change to realise the directorates model.

In the end, the structure should permit the clinician to participate in the allocation and monitoring of resources in clinical care.

In summary, the common goal of doctors and managers is to provide quality care. The important thing to realise is that we can approach care with a focus on quality and together use that approach to gain a greater understanding of each other.

17

Developing Doctors' Management Skills

Austin L. Leahy, Teresa O'Hara and *David Bouchier-Hayes*

Introduction

Doctors are managers. By definition, they are responsible for the output of others, and as professionals their effectiveness is dependent on the involvement of others. Consequently, doctors have increasingly recognised the management role within their practice. Business and management issues are an increasing part of a doctor's working day (Leider and Bard, 1994).

In the 21st century, full-time involvement of doctors in management will be a legitimate career choice (Guthrie, 1988). Increasingly, doctors will be organised into clinical directorates and this will create an opportunity for more clinical directors. Also, doctors will become involved in the management of hospitals, health boards and the health system in general. Current experience in the United States demonstrates a perceived need by doctors in full-time management for management development (Alberts, 1995). This is understandable, as doctors in management positions may find themselves regarded as enthusiastic amateurs by general managers. In view of this, there has been an increasing number entering Master of Business Administration (MBA) programmes. Anders (1994) has reported that 40 per cent of doctors in full-time management in the United States either have an MBA or are entered in an MBA programme.

In the next century, there will be an increasing emphasis on management development in medical education, from an undergraduate level through to a postgraduate level. The recognition that interpersonal skills can be developed, such as communication and negotiation, have led to incorporation of these subjects in undergraduate education. Increasingly, doctors in training are expected to provide added value by demonstrating management competence. The question is therefore no longer whether doctors need to develop management skills, but is rather which management skills should they develop and how should these be developed.

WHICH SKILLS?

Many of the skills which we acquire as doctors are also good management skills. It must be recognised, however, that doctors do not automatically make good managers. There are many aspects of a clinician's work which would seem to be at odds with the work of a manager. Clinicians are generally reactive, in contrast to managers, who must be proactive. The clinician values independence and often acts autonomously. In contrast, the manager must be participative, with the ability to build teams and orchestrate the expertise of others. The clinician's most sacred task is clinical independence, within which the role as patient advocate is paramount. The manager, on the other hand, must consider the competing demands of groups of patients.

A good doctor will quite correctly compete with colleagues for the advancement of an individual patient's needs. Managers seek to create a co-operative environment for the maximisation of resources for all patients. Put simply, the challenge in management development is to improve the doctor's ability to be a team player.

Physicians require a number of personal management skills. It is recognised that medicine can be particularly stressful and stress management skills are easily developed on courses. Time management is also invaluable, as are other personal skills such as assertiveness training.

Arguably, the most basic tool of medicine is negotiation. In all aspects of a physician's involvement with patients and surrounding professionals, negotiation is key. Negotiation may be as simple as discussing a treatment regimen with a patient, or as complex as debating budgets at Board level. Communication is also important and in particular physicians need to learn the art of proper delegation. Too often, delegation is seen as an opportunity to dump jobs rather than an opportunity to develop staff and achieve an added value by the input of others.

Surveys of physicians always highlight the economic area as an area in which doctors feel that they need to develop their knowledge. It is increasingly important that doctors are equipped to become involved in departmental budgeting. Hillman et al. (1985) found that doctors felt that financial analysis, cost accounting, economics, decision analysis, marketing and strategic planning were the other areas where physicians perceived a need for development. The challenge for educationalists is to find suitable educational initiatives for the widespread imparting of management skills which will be necessary for the 21st century.

MANAGEMENT DEVELOPMENT AT THE ROYAL COLLEGE OF SURGEONS IN IRELAND

Since 1990, the RCSI has developed a full range of courses which go a long way towards filling the need for management development for physicians.

At an undergraduate level, students are taught negotiation and communication, stress and time management, and the basics of team dynamics. Specific instruction with regard to the nature of hospitals and the structure of the health system are also given. In many ways, the emphasis on involving the student in teams during clinical training is the most practical management opportunity.

Since 1990, introductory courses in management have been aimed at non-consultant hospital doctors. These are directly supported by the Department of Health. They are principally aimed at providing a foundation in management education, to develop positive attitudes towards management, and where possible to develop management skills. Over 200 doctors have completed this course to date. In the 21st century, this type of course should be mandatory for all doctors involved in the health system. As well as the benefit they will provide to patients, they should also help introduce efficiencies into the system.

Since 1993, the RCSI has offered a Diploma in Management for medical doctors, with the co-operation of the Institute of Public Administration (IPA). This course involves 150 hours of tuition, the completion of two assignments and one project. The emphasis on this course is on offering learning opportunities which are very much rooted in the Irish health system. The courses have succeeded not only because of the considerable amount of time that both the RCSI and the IPA have put into establishing the courses, but also because of the support of the Department of Health. This commitment has been stated in the strategy document *Shaping a Healthier Future — A Strategy for Effective Healthcare in the 1990s.*

It cannot be stressed enough that the principal aim of courses such as the Diploma in Management for Medical Doctors is to make doctors more effective in their current workplace. While the diploma will clearly be helpful to doctors who are embarking on a more formal management role, this is not its primary purpose. A total of 215 doctors have completed the Diploma in Management successfully, and a much greater need for these type of courses can be anticipated in the next century.

Since February 1996, the College has offered an MBA in association with University College Dublin (UCD), whose MBA is recognised to be one of the best on offer in Europe. This degree is aimed at health service professionals in general, and therefore it is particularly useful for doctors who are moving into management positions. The learning environment is very interactive, which allows doctors to benefit from the exchange they can have with other healthcare professionals. The course is offered on a part-time basis over two years, which allows doctors to continue working in their current position.

In the next century, the option of management as a speciality within medicine will become viable. It is inevitable that more and more doctors will seek out an MBA very much in the way professional qualifications are sought out by surgeons, physicians and obstetricians at present.

CONCLUSION

The next century will see a huge increase in numbers enrolling on management development programmes. The previous Minister for Health, Mr Noonan (1996), has acknowledged this. The need for widespread management training requires us to recognise both the content and also the form of development necessary for doctors.

A great deal of the type of management development required has been piloted at the RCSI in partnership with the IPA and UCD. In the next century, there will be a great increase in the number of courses and also greater integration of medical and non-medical health service personnel. We may also see the development of newer educational formats such as fellowships, which allow physicians to take a mid-career break.

The largest constraint on the development of management training in Ireland for doctors is financial. The Department of Health needs to recognise its financial responsibility with respect to the development of sufficient courses. The funding of management development is expensive and it is unrealistic to expect doctors to fund this sort of education themselves. More importantly, the cost of management education would be recouped many times in savings to the system.

The RCSI sees management and business training very much as a continuum beginning at undergraduate level and proceeding into postgraduate development. In that regard, management development is as much about health as it is about management.

References

Alberts, W. (1995), "Business and Management Training for Physicians: CME or Third Degree", *Chest*, Vol. 108, pp. 1711–7.

Anders, G. (1994), "A New Breed of MDs Add MBA to Vitae", *Wall Street Journal*, 27 September, B1, B10.

Guthrie, M. (1988), "Why Physicians Move into Management" in W. Curry (ed.), *New Leadership in Health Care Management: the Physician Executive*, Tampa, FL: American College of Physician Executives, pp. 45–9.

Hillman, A.L., D.B. Nash, W.L. Kissick, et al. (1985), "Managing the Medical-Industrial Complex", *New England Journal of Medicine*, pp. 511–15.

Leider, H.L., M. Bard (1994), "Leadership in Managed Care Organisations: the Role of the Physician Manager" in D.B. Nash (ed.), *The Physician's Guide to Manage Care*, Gaithesbury, MD: Aspen Publishers, pp. 63–9.

Noonan, M. (1996), "What They Don't Teach You in Medical School", *Irish Medical Journal*, Vol. 89, pp. 4–5.

INDEX